Basic Concepts of
Health Care
Human Resource
Management

Nancy J. Niles
Department of Business Administration
Lander University
Greenwood, SC

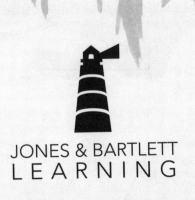

JONES & BARTLETT
LEARNING

World Headquarters
Jones & Bartlett Learning
5 Wall Street
Burlington, MA 01803
978-443-5000
info@jblearning.com
www.jblearning.com

Jones & Bartlett Learning books and products are available through most bookstores and online booksellers. To contact Jones & Bartlett Learning directly, call 800-832-0034, fax 978-443-8000, or visit our website, www.jblearning.com.

Substantial discounts on bulk quantities of Jones & Bartlett Learning publications are available to corporations, professional associations, and other qualified organizations. For details and specific discount information, contact the special sales department at Jones & Bartlett Learning via the above contact information or send an email to specialsales@jblearning.com.

Production Credits

Publisher: Michael Brown

Managing Editor: Maro Gartside

Editorial Assistant: Chloe Falivene

Production Manager: Tracey McCrea

Production Assistant: Alyssa Lawrence

Senior Marketing Manager: Sophie Fleck Teague

Manufacturing and Inventory Control Supervisor: Amy Bacus

Composition: Laserwords Private Limited, Chennai, India

Cover Design: Michael O'Donnell

Cover Image: © SurlyaPhoto/ShutterStock, Inc.

Printing and Binding: Edwards Brothers Malloy

Cover Printing: Edwards Brothers Malloy

To order this product, use ISBN: 978-1-4496-5329-3

Library of Congress Cataloging-in-Publication Data
Niles, Nancy J.
  Basic concepts of health care human resource management / Nancy J. Niles.
      p. ; cm.
  Includes index.
  ISBN 978-1-4496-2782-9 (pbk.) — ISBN 1-4496-2782-X (pbk.)
  I. Title.
  [DNLM: 1. Personnel Management. 2. Health Personnel—organization & administration. W 80]

610.7306'9—dc23

2011045481

6048

Printed in the United States of America
16 15 14 13 12   10 9 8 7 6 5 4 3 2 1

Contents

PART III ■ Training and Developing the Organization   139

CHAPTER 5 ■ Careers in Health Care   141

CHAPTER 6 ■ Employee Benefits   177

CHAPTER 7 ■ Training, Developing, and Motivating Healthcare Employees 209

PART IV ■ Employee Relations 235

CHAPTER 8 ■ Labor Unions and Health Care 237

Preface

I have been teaching human resource management for many years. Prior to teaching, I was in management. I realized as I managed employees how important human resource management is to the success of an organization. I think any human resource management course should be a core course for all managers, regardless of industry. If you can't manage your employees, your organization will not be successful, plain and simple. Yet it continues to amaze me how often a human resource department is located in the basement of a building, far from senior management.

Although larger organizations have established human resource management departments that managers can utilize, smaller organizations may not have an HR department; therefore, general management should be comfortable with human resource management activities. This textbook will provide information that both general managers and human resource managers can apply to the healthcare industry. The textbook is organized as follows:

■ Part 1: Introduction

This textbook provides a glimpse into the importance of human resource management (HRM) in all aspects of healthcare organizations. Each chapter discusses HRM and its role in many different aspects of healthcare management. The following is a summary of each of the chapters of this textbook as they relate to HRM.

Chapter 1

This introductory chapter emphasizes the important role that human resource management activities play in the operations of a healthcare organization. It is fascinating that human resource management activities were observed as early as 2000 B.C. Human resources can be applied to any activity of the operations of an organization, regardless of the industry. The role of HRM is briefly discussed in this chapter on organizational activities, including legal and ethical issues of the treatment, health and safety of employees and patients, careers in health care, labor unions in health care, job analysis and design, recruiting and selecting employees, employee benefits, training and motivating employees, and terminating employees. Strategic planning, including labor budget and forecasting, is addressed because of the contribution of HRM to successful strategic planning. Emerging and current trends in human resource management are also discussed. The increased diversity of the patient and employee, the effect of technology and the globalization of the economy on healthcare delivery, the new trend of medical tourism, and the increased focus on accountability in the delivery of services and teamwork education are exciting changes in health care, which ultimately will improve patient care. All of these major changes have an impact on how human resource management assists with these organizational changes.

Chapter 2

A healthcare manager must be familiar with the different federal and state laws that affect the healthcare industry. The HRM department must provide training for all employees to ensure they understand the seriousness of violating the law as well as the differences between civil and criminal law and the penalties that may be imposed for breaking those laws. Federal and state laws and policies have been implemented to protect both the healthcare provider and the healthcare consumer. New laws have been passed and older laws have been amended to reflect needed changes regarding health care and the protection of its participants. If an organization and its employees perform research, Institutional Review Board (IRB) training must be implemented to ensure that ethical guidelines are followed when performing research on humans. Human resource departments and managers must discuss ethics in the workplace and develop a code of ethics for all employees to understand and follow. An aspect of ethical behavior is the issue of workplace bullying, which is common in the healthcare industry. Codes of ethics provide a standard for operation so that all participants understand that if they do not adhere to this code, there may be negative consequences. Because of continued legal changes, HRM offers training on a routine basis. Ethical training must also be offered on a continual basis. Employees at all levels are faced with healthcare ethical dilemmas.

■ Part II: Staffing the Organization

Chapter 3

Evaluating the workflow of any organization is the first step to developing jobs that ensure the desired outputs of an organization are produced. Once the workflow is analyzed, the next step is to create jobs for individuals who will be employed by the organization and who will be responsible for producing the output of the organization. Prior to creating the jobs, a job analysis must be performed to determine which type of activities an employee will need to perform within a certain position in the organization. Job analysis is the foundation of human resource management because it is required before an organization recruits individuals for specific jobs. At the conclusion of a job analysis, a written job description and specifications are developed that outline the responsibilities, skills, and experience needed to perform the job successfully.

How the jobs are designed is an important part of development. The design must ensure the health and safety of the employees through ergonomics, that the work is performed efficiently, and that the employees are motivated to perform at a high level. Motivational job designs include flextime, job sharing, job enlargement, enrichment, rotation, and telework.

The same process must be performed if the organization decides to alter the way a service is being offered. For example, if electronic medical records will be implemented in a healthcare facility, it is necessary to determine the current workflow patterns and then redesign the projected workflow to accommodate the new technology. If an organization is diligent in these job processes, analysis and design will help the organization perform at its highest level.

Chapter 4

An organization should plan a systematic recruitment process to ensure that the appropriate candiates apply for positions. Organizations can recruit both internally and externally to the organization. Regardless of the recruitment method, the organization must assess the effectiveness of the types of recruitment methods chosen. Once the recruitment process has been completed, the next step is to select the appropriate candiates for the organization. This step consists of interviews and, in some instances, tests that assess aptitude, attitude, honesty, and personality. These procesess must be legally defensible, which means that the processes must be objective and fair to all applicants. Human resource management plays a huge role in these processes in order to ensure that the most qualified applicants are hired for the organization.

■ Part III: Training and Developing the Organization

Chapter 5

Healthcare personnel represent one of the largest labor forces in the United States. This chapter provides an overview of the different types of employees in the healthcare industry. Some of them require many years of education; however, some of these positions can be achieved through 1–2 year programs. According to the Centers for Disease Control and Prevention 2012 statistics, health care is the one of the fastest growing sectors of the U.S. economy, representing 12 million workers. The healthcare industry will continue to evolve as the United States' trends in demographics, disease, and public health patterns change. More occupations and professions will develop because of these trends. The major trend that will influence the healthcare industry is the aging of the U.S. population. The Bureau of Labor Statistics predicts that half of the next decades' fastest growing jobs will be in the healthcare industry. As healthcare costs continue to increase, cost-cutting measures will be the focus while continuing to provide quality health care.

Chapter 6

It is the responsibility of HRM personnel to ensure that legally mandated employee benefits—social security, unemployment insurance and workmen's compensation, and family and medical leave—are implemented correctly. In addition, there are several employee benefits that employers can offer to employees that can be used as a recruitment and/or retention tool. Employees expect employers to provide medical insurance, including dental and vision plans, and vacation, sick leave, and retirement plans. However, employers have the opportunity to offer other benefits such as education reimbursement, child or elder care services, or flexible work schedules. Employers may consider a cafeteria plan which enables employees to select which benefits are best suited for their lifestyle. Employers should survey their employees and their competition to determine the best type of benefits package that would motivate and retain quality employees. Establishing a quality benefits package would also be an excellent recruitment tool. Human resource management can collaborate with management to ensure that the best recruitment packages are offered to quality candidates.

Chapter 7

The goal of healthcare organizations is to provide quality of care to their patients. Nurses, physicians, and other healthcare providers have direct contact with patients. There are also different types of healthcare employees that provide indirect care to patients. Laboratory technologists and technicians have a major role in diagnosing disease, assessing the impact of interventions, and applying highly technical procedures, but they may never see the patients directly.

Regardless of their role, underperforming employees could risk the lives of their patients. Research on high performing organizations, including healthcare organizations, reveals that employees are motivated to perform well by the quality of work environment. A quality work environment includes initiatives such as employee empowerment, training and career development programs for employees, pay for performance, management transparency, and support and work-life balance (Lowe, 2002). This chapter discusses different motivational theories and organizational strategies to motivate employee performance.

■ Part IV: Employee Relations

Chapter 8

Regardless of the industry, unions are formed because employees are dissatisfied with their jobs. Either the wages are too low or the working conditions are poor.

As healthcare expenditures continue to increase, healthcare reform will continue to focus on cost reduction. Managed care models targeted labor costs, which resulted in disgruntled physicians and nurses because they were worried about the quality of patient care (Schraeder & Friedman, 2002). Nurses formed unions because they were more concerned with quality working conditions to ensure patient care than wages. Residents and interns were also concerned with working conditions because of the traditional long hours they endure while training. Establishing a union resulted in limited working hours for them. Allied health professional unions have been established to ensure that fair wages are being applied in their industry. It has been difficult for physician unions to become more powerful because so many physicians are self-employed and therefore excluded from union membership. However, there are exceptional health systems, such as the Cleveland Clinic, which are excellent to their physician employees (Romano, 2001). With the advent of the healthcare reform legislation and the reduction of reimbursement of physician services to Medicare and Medicaid patients, there may be more of a reason to organize. Over the past 5 years, unions won 70% of healthcare organizing efforts with New York, California, and Illinois representing nearly 50% of the total elections (By the Numbers, 2009). In 2009, there were 11 strikes, which affected 2,600 workers, or 238 workers per strike, which is low. In 2010, there were seven strikes involving 14,000 workers, or 2,000 workers per strike (Commis, 2010).

Regardless of their goals, union formation in the healthcare industry is characterized by the merging of several unions to increase their voice in dealing with their employers. Large unions such as the American Federation of Teachers (AFT) and the Service Employees International Union (SEIU) have established separate legal entities that represent healthcare issues. Although union membership in the United States has declined over the past decades, union membership in the healthcare industry has increased.

Chapter 9

Terminating an employee is one of the most difficult responsibilities for a manager because it influences the individual's life and livelihood. If you have to terminate an employee, it may indicate that the organization's hiring process is not adequate. However, there are many hiring guidelines to ensure that the termination process is fair and legally defensible. The following are activities that HRM should be involved in when dealing with such a difficult employee issue:

1. Educating employees on employment law and company policies.
2. Communicating verbally and in writing the expectations the organization has of the employee's performance.
3. Enforcing labor laws equally to all employees to ensure there are no issues with discrimination of protected classes.

4. Establishing routine performance appraisals of all employees.
5. Providing employee feedback.
6. Establishing a termination deadline.
7. Establishing exit interviews for all employees.

■ Part V: Long-Term Planning in HR

Chapter 10

There are many current trends influencing healthcare human resource management: the increasing diversity of the workforce, the globalization of health care, increased use of technology and its impact on the healthcare system, and the focus on teamwork and quality patient care.

There is an increased diversity of employees and patients. These changing demographics can also be linked to the increased globalization of health care. There is more U.S. patient circulation internationally because of the high costs of health care, which results in patients finding treatments outside the United States. Additionally, due to the lack of primary physicians and nurses nationally, more international employees are being hired. The use of technology in health care continues to increase. The federal focus on the implementation of electronic health records for patient information requires more training for employees. There is also a focus of teamwork in health care, which requires different professional development for employees. This chapter discusses these current trends and provides recommendations to healthcare organizations to develop training programs for their employees to ensure they are comfortable with their changing environment.

Chapter 11

In any organization, it is necessary to develop both short-term and long-term plans to ensure the organization will successfully continue. Managers typically focus on short-term goals through their daily activities and monthly planning. What often eludes managers is the long-term planning needed to determine future activities of the organization. Long-term planning or strategic management is necessary to ensure the longevity of the organization. Developing a mission and vision statement for the organization provides a focus for the employees to understand what the organization is doing and what their future plans are. With any mission and vision statement, the role of HRM is simple: ensure there are employees in place that have the skills and knowledge to achieve the mission and vision of the organization. Recruiting, training, and retaining the appropriate employees is a fundamental HRM process. It is important to emphasize that HRM is an administrative function of an organization; however, when it is involved in strategic planning, the HRM process is altered because its focus is not daily operations but long term.

There is a continuing labor shortage in the healthcare industry, and projections indicate the shortage may continue for years. Therefore, in healthcare strategic management, HRM plays an integral role in strategic planning to address workforce needs and projected shortages. As part of strategic planning, quality programs are implemented to provide guidelines for quality control. These quality programs are also integrated with human resource management. Finally, budgeting for these long-term needs must also be addressed. This chapter discusses the concepts of strategic management as they apply to healthcare organizations and the role of human resource management in strategic management.

Acknowledgments

As always, my mother, Joyce Robinson, continues to inspire me as my role model.

My husband, Donnie, who is my biggest supporter and who encouraged me to write another textbook.

Kudos to my nephew, Aaron Robinson, who continues to follow his musical dreams!

Thank you as always to Mike Brown, Publisher, Maro Gartside, Managing Editor, and Chloe Falivene, Editorial Assistant for providing me with invaluable support and advice on this project. Thank you also to Alyssa Lawrence, Production Assistant, for her patience with my chronic editing.

About the Author

Nancy J. Niles is an Associate Professor teaching undergraduate business and healthcare management classes in the AACSB accredited Department of Business Administration at Lander University in Greenwood, South Carolina. She became very interested in healthcare issues after spending nearly five years with the U.S. Peace Corps in Senegal, West Africa. Her graduate education has focused on health policy and management. She received her PhD from the University of Illinois at Urbana-Champaign, Master of Public Health from Tulane University's School of Public Health and Tropical Medicine, and a Master of Science with emphasis in healthcare administration and a Master of Business Administration from the University of Maryland's University College. Her first undergraduate textbook, *Basics of the U.S. Health Care System*, was also published by Jones & Bartlett Learning.

Introduction

What Is Human Resource Management?

The student will be able to:

- Discuss the history of human resource management.
- Define human resource management.
- Identify four applications of human resource management to healthcare organizations.
- Examine the importance of human resource management to organizations.
- Assess the impact of Frederick W. Taylor on managing employees.
- Analyze the impact of the Hawthorne studies on motivating employees.

DID YOU KNOW THAT?

- The Chinese and Greeks used employee screening and apprenticeship programs in 2000 B.C.
- It is the legal responsibility of the employer to provide a safe and healthy work environment.
- The healthcare industry employs more than 3% of the U.S. workforce.
- Employee benefits are considered incentives to recruit and retain employees.
- In 1900, the B.F. Goodrich Company was the first to establish a human resource management department.

■ Introduction

Human resource management is defined as a system of activities and strategies that focus on successfully managing employees at all levels of an organization to achieve organizational goals (Byars & Rue, 2006). Employees are the human resources of an organization and its most valuable asset. To be successful, an organization must make employee productivity a major goal. The level of productivity can vary depending on the skill levels the employees demonstrate in their jobs and the satisfaction levels of the employees with the organization and their jobs. To develop a high-performance and effective workforce, the organization should use human resource management input in the following organizational areas:

1. Establishment of a legal and ethical management system
2. Job analysis and job design
3. Recruitment and selection
4. Healthcare career opportunities
5. Distribution of employee benefits
6. Employee motivation
7. Negotiations with organized labor
8. Employee terminations
9. Determination of emerging and future trends in health care
10. Strategic planning

■ Major Milestones of Human Resource Management

At what point in history did the concept of human resource management emerge (Table 1.1)? During prehistoric times, there existed consistent methods for selection of tribal leaders. The practice of safety and health while hunting was passed on from generation to generation. From 2000 B.C. to 1500 B.C., the Chinese used employee-screening techniques, and the Greeks used an apprentice system (History of Human Resource Management, 2010). These actions recognized the need to select and train individuals for jobs.

During the late 1700s and early 1800s, because of the rapid industrialization of Great Britain, the United States evolved from an agricultural nation to an industrial nation. British factories were being built, and innovative manufacturing processes were being developed. The United States benefitted from this progress as British immigrants brought their new knowledge to the United States. Because of this **Industrial Revolution**, there developed a separate class of managers and employees in the factories (The Emergence of Modern Industrialism, 2010). **Labor unions** were established from 1790 to 1820. These membership labor organizations represented different types of skilled employees, such as printers or carpenters, to ensure that these employees were treated fairly by management. Labor unions focused on job security, fair wages, and shorter working hours for employees (Byars & Rue, 2006). This dramatic change in the U.S. economy emphasized the need for a system in the workplace to manage both employees and management—the human resources of these new types of organizations. During this period, labor unions became powerful advocates for employee

Table 1.1 Major Milestones of Human Resource Management Development in the United States

2000–1500 B.C.	Chinese use employee-screening techniques.
	Greeks use an apprentice system.
1700 to early 1800	U.S. evolved from agricultural nation to industrial nation.
	Great Britain experienced rapid industrialization.
	British immigrants brought industrialization knowledge to the U.S. A new U.S. labor system established a division of labor: management and employees.
1790–1820	Labor unions were established to protect employees' rights.
1900	B.F. Goodrich Company established the first HR department.
1902	National Cash Register established an HR department to handle employee issues.
1911	Frederick W. Taylor: Scientific management principles established differential pay system.
1913	U.S. Department of Labor was established to promote welfare of employees.
1920–1930	Hawthorne studies: Increased productivity by changing the physical work environment of the employees.
1935	Social Security Act was passed, which created "old age" insurance for those of retirement age. Through payroll taxes, employees pay a portion of their wages to contribute to the fund.
1938	Fair Labor Standards Act of 1938 established federal minimum wage laws.
1960–1980	Equal Pay Act of 1963, Civil Rights Act of 1964, Occupational Health and Safety Act of 1970, and Pregnancy Discrimination Act of 1978. These Acts focused on employee discrimination and safety.
1990	Americans with Disabilities Act of 1990 and Older Workers Benefit Protection Act of 1990 prohibit discrimination against disabled workers and workers greater than 40 years of age.

(continues)

Table 1.1 (Continued)

2008–2009	Genetic Information Nondiscrimination Act of 2008 and the Lilly Ledbetter Fair Pay Act of 2009: Legislation prohibiting genetic testing and compensation discrimination.
2010	Patient Protection and Affordable Care Act of 2010 (PPACA): Controversial legislation that requires individuals to purchase health insurance by 2014. Contested by several states for its constitutionality, provisions of the Act will be reviewed by the Supreme Court most likely in 2012.

rights, although there were many court skirmishes attempting to mitigate the power of unions over the decades.

From 1950 to 1970, union membership represented more than 25% of the U.S. workforce. From 1980 to 1999, as the U.S. economy focused less on manufacturing and evolved into a service economy, union membership declined (Mathis & Jackson, 2006). Although union membership has since continued to decline, labor unions can be regarded as the predecessors of human resource management departments. The goal of both is the equitable treatment of employees by management.

In 1900, the B.F. Goodrich Company pioneered the establishment of an employee department to address labor concerns. In 1902, National Cash Register also formed a separate department to handle employee issues such as wages and grievances (History of Human Resource Management, 2010). More companies eventually followed their lead in human resource management.

A labor shortage existed in the early 20th century, thus management focused on increasing the productivity of its employees. In 1911, **Frederick W. Taylor** promoted scientific management through four principles:

1. Evaluate a task by dissecting its components.
2. Select employees that had the appropriate skills for a task.
3. Provide workers with incentives and training to do a task.
4. Use science to plan how workers perform their jobs (Kinicki & Williams, 2008).

Taylor developed a differential pay system that rewarded workers who performed at a higher level. This type of human resource management is still used today.

Because of the economic revolution in the United States, a federal agency, the **U.S. Department of Labor,** was established in 1913 by President Taft. Its mission was and is to promote the welfare of working people and their work conditions. By the end of World War I, the Department of Labor had established policies to ensure that fair wages and work conditions existed so that human resources, the employees, were treated fairly (Department of Labor, 2010).

In the 1920s, a Harvard research group implemented the **"Hawthorne studies,"** which focused on changing the physical work environments of employees to assess any changes in their work habits. The results indicated an increase in productivity, as workers believed that management was concerned about their welfare, which improved their productivity. Although these experiments were eventually criticized for having a poor research design, they illustrated the importance of management treating employees well as an impetus to improved worker performance (Kinicki & Williams, 2008). The Fair Labor Standards Act of 1938, enforced by the U.S. Department of Labor, established federal minimum wage standards, child labor laws, and increased wages for overtime. Both laws and management theory established the precedent for human resource management today.

Recent Milestones of Human Resource Management

During the 1960s and 1970s, legislation such as the Equal Pay Act of 1963, the Civil Rights Act of 1964, the Occupational Safety and Health Act of 1970, and the Pregnancy Discrimination Act of 1978 required employers to recognize employee rights. During the 1980s and 1990s, legislation such as the Americans with Disabilities Act of 1990 and the Older Workers Benefit Protection Act of 1990 further supported employee rights. Recently, legislation such as the Genetic Information Nondiscrimination Act of 2008 and the Lilly Ledbetter Fair Pay Act of 2009 continued to focus on employment discrimination. The Patient Protection and Affordability Act of 2010 goal, although controversial, was to increase the number of individuals who will have health care insurance.

■ The Role of Human Resources in Healthcare Organizations

The role of human resource management is that of a partnership between the human resources (HR) department and management regardless of the organizational type. Most HR departments have similar responsibilities. The HR and management partnership is unique in the healthcare industry because many healthcare organizations have a dual administrative structure of clinical managers and health services managers that supervise two distinct groups of employees with different responsibilities and different training needs. For example, clinical managers have training or experience in a specific clinical area and, accordingly, have more specific responsibilities than do generalists or health services managers. For example, directors of physical therapy are experienced physical therapists, nurse managers have nursing degrees, but most health service managers have a bachelor's degree or master's degree in health services (BLS, 2011).

According to Zingheim and Schuster (2002), there are steps that an organization can take to foster a relationship between the HR department and senior management:

1. Treat HR employees as internal consultants to the organization who can provide recommendations about employee relations.
2. Ensure that management actively collaborates with HR employees, which includes inviting HR management to strategic planning meetings.
3. Ensure that HR provides extensive training to all employees on a routine basis.
4. Both HR and management should participate in an HR audit to assess the state of the organization. Turnover rates, incentive plans, diversity rates, and strategic planning activities should be continuously reviewed to ensure the organization is performing at a high level.

The following sections of this chapter describe specific workplace issues where the role of HR management is integrated to ensure that these issues are addressed throughout an organization.

Legal, Ethical, and Safety Issues in Health Care

Employees at all levels should have an understanding of basic legal and ethical principles that affect the work environment, particularly in the healthcare industry. The legal relationship between the organization and the consumer—the healthcare provider and the patient—is the foundational relationship of all healthcare activities. Ethical behaviors, which are considered actions that are the right thing to do, not simply what is required by law, must also be addressed because the healthcare industry is fraught with difficult situations that involve ethical dilemmas.

Federal and state laws have been passed and policies have been implemented to protect both the healthcare provider and the healthcare consumer. The passage of new laws and amendments of older laws reflect needed changes to protect healthcare participants. For example, if research is performed by the organization and its employees, training must be implemented to ensure that ethical guidelines are followed when performing human research . A recent employee issue is that of workplace bullying, which is common in the healthcare industry. Workplace bullying awareness training is needed to address this unethical issue (Minding the Workplace, 2011). It is the role of the HR department and management to train employees at all levels regarding employment-related legislation. It is also the responsibility of HR and management to create an ethical organizational culture by providing ethics training and codes of ethics.

Another major employment issue is that of a safe working environment. According to the federal **Occupational Safety and Health Administration (OSHA)**, it is the responsibility of the organization to monitor and ensure a safe and healthy work environment for employees (OSHA, 2011). Healthcare employees are exposed to toxic chemicals, contaminated blood, bacteria, and radiation. Hospitals, laboratories, physicians' and other healthcare providers' offices, and skilled nursing facilities require constant surveillance by OSHA to monitor workplace standards. As part of health and safety, the **Joint Commission** (formerly the Joint Commission on Accreditation of Healthcare Organizations [JCAHO]), also reviews health and safety standards for both patients and employees (Minding the Workplace, 2011). In collaboration with HR departments, OSHA provides training and educational materials to inform employees about the dangers of the workplace.

Job Analysis and Design

When starting or expanding any organization, the first goal is to determine its overall mission. If the mission is long-term care, for example, the first major decision is to decide how the work or tasks will flow through the organization to accomplish this goal. This process also applies to existing healthcare organizations if they decide to change their services. For example, healthcare organizations have integrated technology into their operations, such as the implementation of electronic patient health records. This type of major transition would require a review of the workflow to ensure this new activity would be successful. Evaluating the workflow of any organization is the first step in job development to produce the desired outputs of an organization. The second step in job development is job analysis.

The HR department is responsible for performing job analyses to assess the workflow of the organization. **Job analysis** is a process of determining the different tasks that are associated with a specific job (Dessler, 2012). It is the foundation of HR management. Job analysis is the tool for organizations to understand what type of staffing and training is required to ensure the high performance of employees. Job analysis enables the organization to develop job descriptions and specifications to recruit individuals that have specific knowledge, skills, and abilities for these jobs. The next step in the process of job development is job design.

Job design defines how tasks are performed and the types of tasks that are part of a job (Mathis & Jackson, 2006). Job design can be considered a retention strategy to encourage employee satisfaction. In health care, job design is less flexible than in other industries because many job responsibilities have legal restrictions and standards. However, teamwork is commonly used in the healthcare industry and can have some flexibility with its structure. **Team designs** such as functional teams, project teams, self-directed teams, task forces, and virtual teams are used in healthcare organizations. Job design in teams can be an important tool to ensure that teams fulfill their designated goals. In addition, **job schedule redesign,** such as flextime or compressed work schedules, may be an incentive for employee satisfaction and motivation (Byars & Rue, 2006). Once job analyses and job design are performed, the next step is to recruit the best employees for these jobs.

Recruitment, Selection, and Retention

The HR department is responsible for collaboration with management to ensure that the recruitment and selection process is **legally defensible**, which means the process is systematic and fair in order to objectively and fairly recruit and select potential employees. A legally defensible process must adhere to legal standards. HR collaborates with management to retain the best employees for the organization. **Recruitment** consists of any activity that focuses on attracting the appropriate candidates to fulfill job openings in the organization. Once candidates are identified, the next step is the **selection** process, which identifies the best employees for the organization (Noe, Hollenbeck, Gerhart & Wright, 2011). The selection process must abide by appropriate legal standards. Once an organization selects the preferred candidate, the organization should create a culture to retain its valued employees. Employee turnover costs industries millions of dollars annually. Recruitment, selection, and retention are very important in the healthcare industry. The nursing profession, often considered the backbone of health care, has experienced labor shortages for several years. This shortage is expected to continue for several years. There also continues to be a shortage of physicians in rural communities and in certain urban areas; thus, these two professions are a focus of many recruitment, selection, and retention strategies by HR and management.

Healthcare Career Opportunities

The healthcare industry is one of the largest employers in the United States, employing more than 3% of the U.S. workforce. There are approximately 200 health occupations and professions and a workforce of more than 14 million healthcare workers. Between 2005 and 2030, the 65 years and older demographic will increase from 6% to 10% of the total population, which will increase pressure on the healthcare system (National Center for Health Statistics, 2008). Because of the aging of our population, the Bureau of Labor Statistics indicates that health care will generate more than nearly 4 million new jobs through 2014 (High Growth Industry Profile: Health Care, 2007). When we think of healthcare providers, one automatically thinks of physicians and nurses. However, the healthcare industry is comprised of many different health service professionals. The healthcare industry includes dentists, optometrists, psychologists, chiropractors, podiatrists, non-physician practitioners, administrators, and allied health professionals. **Allied health professionals** are an integral component of this industry, as they provide a range of essential healthcare services that complement the services provided by physicians and nurses. Allied health professionals constitute 60% of the U.S. healthcare workforce (Shi & Singh, 2008). There are many opportunities for healthcare employees to have a long-term career in this industry. An excellent HR department provides career development guidance for employees.

Healthcare Employee Benefits

Employee benefits are a typical responsibility of the HR department. HR personnel educate employees about employee benefits and administer these benefits programs. Social security, unemployment insurance, workers' compensation, and unpaid family and medical leave are employee benefits required by law or **mandatory benefits.** Employee **voluntary benefits**, which are not required by law, such as retirement plans, paid leave, and different types of family care can be considered a recruitment tool because they can attract qualified candidates (Mathis & Jackson, 2006). Most full-time employees expect healthcare benefits, but there are other benefits that are attractive to employees, which motivate them to remain with an organization. Some potential employees may sacrifice salary expectations in exchange for benefits such as flexible scheduling, so benefits can play a role in attracting the right employees. Offering benefits that are attractive to employees may result in lower turnover for the organization.

Motivating Healthcare Employees

The goal of healthcare organizations is to provide the highest quality of patient care. The development of incentives such as work–life balance programs and employee career programs is an example of how HR can play an integral role in a high-performance organization. Nurses, physicians, and other healthcare providers have direct contact with patients. However, there are categories of healthcare employees that may provide indirect care to patients. Laboratory technologists and technicians or clinical laboratory technologists and technicians have a major role in diagnosing disease, assessing the impact of interventions, and applying highly technical procedures but may never see the patients directly. Regardless of the direct or indirect roles of providing health care, employees that are not performing at a high level could risk the lives of patients.

Research on high-performing organizations, including healthcare organizations, reveals that employees are motivated to perform well by the quality of the work environment including employee empowerment, training and career development programs, pay for performance, management transparency, and work–life balance philosophy.

Employee development consists of programs that focus on the expansion of an employee's career. Development programs tend to be long term and are awarded to employees that the organization believes have potential for promotion. **Employee training** programs improve an employee's performance in his or her current job (Dessler, 2012). Training can occur before a new employee starts a job or training can be given to employees during their tenure. Development and training programs can be a source of motivation to employees to improve their performance. Financial incentives can also be a source of motivation to improve employee productivity.

Job redesign such as job enlargement, which expands the number of tasks in a job, and **job enrichment,** which increases the responsibilities of a job, are both motivational strategies. Both of these job redesigns provide a sense of employee empowerment because the employer is recognizing the ability of the employee to increase his or her workload. If an organization provides appropriate individual and group incentives to motivate its employees, the employees may be more inclined to remain with the organization. It is important to create a culture that values the employees and considers them assets.

Labor Unions and Health Care

Labor unions are membership labor organizations formed to protect their members' employee rights. Their main goal is to ensure that management treats its employees fairly. In the early 1900s, the establishment of unions occurred because of the industrialization of the United States and the consequent unfair treatment of employees by management. In 1935, the National Labor Relations Act (NLRA) was passed, which protected the right of workers to form unions, defined unfair labor practices, and established the National Labor Relations Board, which is responsible for NLRA regulatory oversight. It is the only federal union legislation that protects organized labor relations (Gentry, 2008). From 1950 to 1970, union membership represented more than 25% of the U.S. workforce. During the 1980s and 1990s, as the U.S. economy focused less on manufacturing and evolved into a service economy, union membership declined (Mathis & Jackson, 2006). However, service industries such as health care are being targeted by union organizers because they are an untapped source of potential union membership. In 2009, union membership represented 12% of all U.S. workers—a decrease from 24% in 1979. However, union membership in the healthcare industry is increasing slightly. In 2000, 12.9% of healthcare workers were unionized. In 2009, the percentage increased to 13.6% (Davis, 2010). Healthcare unions are increasing in strength, particularly in the nursing sector. In 2007, the Service Employees International Union (SEIU) created a separate national healthcare union, which is the largest healthcare union nationally. SEIU Healthcare represents hospital, nursing, long-term care, and many outpatient facilities. Unions representing physicians are affiliated with SEIU. The California Nurses Association, the National Nurses Organizing Committee, and the United American Nurses merged and created National Nurses United (NNU). The NNU is the largest nurses union in the United States, representing 150,000 members (Malvey, 2010). HR is responsible for engaging in labor negotiations with labor unions.

Terminating Employees

Employment is a legal relationship between an employee and an employer. Both employers and employees have established rights. Employers must provide a safe working environment for their employees. Employees must perform to the best of their ability in accordance with their job descriptions and organizational policies or they may risk being terminated or fired from their jobs. If an organization has a legally defensible, quality hiring process that provides the best employees for the organization, there should be minimal need to terminate many employees. However, in a recent survey of healthcare managers, six reasons for healthcare employee termination were noted: (1) poor performance, (2) ethical misconduct, (3) excessive absences, (4) poor attitude, (5) personality conflicts, and (6) substance abuse (McKinnies, Collins, Collins & Matthews, 2010). Termination of an employee is a very difficult process. Rules and regulations are put in place to ensure that both sides maintain their rights when an employee is terminated. HR is responsible for monitoring an employee termination process.

Current Trends in Health Care

Demographic and Diversity Trends in the Workforce and the Population

Individuals require healthcare services as they age. With the increase in life expectancy in the United States, it is projected that an additional 3 million healthcare jobs will be created by 2018 to care for this population. There is also an increase in the diversity of the U.S. workforce. The projected 2018 workforce is 79% Caucasian, 12% African American, and 9% Asian and other minorities. The number of females in the workplace is expected to reach nearly 47% (Noe et al., 2011). In a 2002 report, the Institute of Medicine indicated there was a dire need to address the racial and ethnic disparities in health services. Research has indicated that there are significant disparities of access to health care based on cultural heritage that must be addressed (Andrulis, 2003). This also influences the diversity of the workforce. It is the responsibility of the HR department and management to develop strategies to respect both aspects of the diverse healthcare industry.

The United States participates in a **global economy**. The U.S. economy has become borderless as a result of information technology. Competing in a global economy has affected the area of human resource management. When companies compete outside their domestic borders, issues of cross-cultural awareness are vital to successful productivity. Employees must be trained in cross-cultural competencies. Because of the shortage of nurses and physicians, foreign healthcare professionals are being hired to work in the United States. In addition, the threat of terrorism has increased over the past decade. If a company decides to operate internationally, it is its responsibility to protect its employees. U.S. citizens are traveling outside the U.S. for medical procedures, which has created a **medical tourism** industry because the procedures are often much less costly overseas. Even with travel costs, international procedures are much less expensive than U.S. medical procedures. U.S. healthcare companies such as Aetna are also expanding their health insurance services overseas to emerging target markets such as India and Brazil's working middle class (Is the Latin American Health, 2011). These trends fall under the purview of human resource management. HR provides extensive cross-cultural training to ensure that diversity is respected in the healthcare environment.

Information Technology Impact

Health or **medical informatics** is the science of computer application that supports clinical and research data in different areas of health care. It is a methodology of how the healthcare industry thinks about patients and how treatments are defined and evolve. **Health information systems** are systems that store, transmit, collect, and retrieve these data (Anderson, Rice & Kominski, 2007). The goal of **health information technology** (HIT) is to manage health data for use by patients/consumers, insurance companies, healthcare providers, healthcare administrators, and any stakeholder that has an interest in health care (Goldstein & Blumenthal, 2008).

HIT affects every aspect of the healthcare industry, and all of the stakeholders in the healthcare industry use HIT. Information technology (IT) has had a tremendous impact on the healthcare industry because it enables rapid documentation of every transaction. When an industry focuses on saving lives, written documentation is required to describe this activity. Computerization of documentation has increased the efficiency of management of healthcare data. The focus of HIT is the national implementation of an electronic patient record. The electronic patient record is the foundation of many IT systems because it will enable systems to share patient information, which will increase the quality and efficiency of health care. A major issue with HIT is sharing and protecting patient information electronically. The HR department uses technology for maintaining electronic files about employees. Human resource management is responsible for protecting the privacy of both employee and patient information.

Teamwork and Accountable Care in Health Care

The Institute of Medicine report *To Err Is Human: Building a Safer Health System* treats the issue of preventable medical errors, which, according to the report, are in part the result of poor teamwork implementation. The report further states that effective teamwork can increase effective patient care. A model of teamwork in health care is the **accountable care organization (ACO)**, which consists of a network of organizations and healthcare providers that offer coordinated care. Their accountability is to improve clinical outcomes for designated populations. If the outcomes are met or exceeded, the group of physicians receives a financial bonus. There may be excessive penalties for not reaching the targets. For example, the Medicare Shared Savings Program will award ACOs rewards for lower patient care costs (Accountable Care Organizations, 2011). The model's assumption is that a group of providers is driven by peer pressure to achieve or exceed its stated objectives. Another form of teamwork is **interprofessional education,** which occurs when two or more professionals from different healthcare sectors engage in a dialogue so they can learn from each other—promoting interprofessional interaction. Interprofessional education promotes effective collaboration during patient care. It is an effective way of providing different perspectives of how to care for a patient within a team.

Pay for Performance

Pay for performance and **value-based purchasing** are terms that describe healthcare payment systems that reward healthcare providers for their **efficiency**, which is defined as providing higher quality care for less cost. They are another form of an accountable care organization. From a healthcare consumer perspective, the stakeholders should hold healthcare providers accountable for both the cost and high quality of their care. Because most health care in the United States historically has been provided by employers, in value-based purchasing, employers select healthcare plans based on demonstrated quality and cost-effectiveness of healthcare delivery (see www.ahrq .gov). Because of the uniqueness of this concept, human resource management plays an active role in training healthcare providers in this type of structure. Regardless of the model chosen, human resource management plays an integral role in the training of these types of programs.

Nursing Home Trends

In 2001, the Robert Wood Johnson Foundation funded a pilot project developed by Dr. Bill Thomas, the **Green House Project,** which is a unique type of nursing home established as a residence that provides services; that is, the concept of being a home to the residents rather than an institution at which to receive care. The home is managed by a team of workers who share the care of the residents including cooking and housekeeping. The daily staff members are certified nursing assistants. All mandated professional personnel such as physicians, nurses, social workers, and dieticians form visiting clinical support teams that assess the elders and supervise their care (Kane, Lum, Cutler, Degenholtz & Yu, 2007). Human resource management can play an active role in training these employees on how to treat their patients in this unique type of environment.

Social Media Communication

Social media is an electronic tool that provides a platform for customer interaction to create public awareness of their business. Facebook, Twitter, and YouTube are examples of social media. It is used increasingly by healthcare organizations not only as a recruiting tool but also as a communications tool for patient engagement, employees, and providers. According to a September 2011 employee survey of IT professionals, administrators, and physicians, 75% use social media for professional purposes in their jobs. The Mayo Clinic and the U.S. Department of Veterans Affairs are exploring ways to use social media for patient engagement including education (Lewis, 2011). Hospitals and academic medical centers are establishing more YouTube channels and Twitter accounts nationwide. Physicians use Twitter to communicate easily and quickly with other physicians. YouTube provides the opportunity to make available brief videos regarding certain points in healthcare education.

Strategic HR Management

The **strategic planning** of an organization consists of long-term goal setting to compete successfully in an industry (Thompson, Strickland & Gamble, 2006). An action plan of how to implement these goals is formulated based on the strengths of the organization. The ultimate goal is to maintain a sustainable competitive advantage over the organization's rivals. As part of this strategic planning process, human resource management plays a role in workforce planning to ensure that there exists the appropriate and adequate labor supply both currently and in the future to satisfy these strategic goals. HR departments have evolved to play an important role in the strategic planning of an organization. This is particularly important because of the continued labor shortage of nurses in the U.S. healthcare system and the geographic maldistribution of physicians who are generalists. Therefore, it may be necessary to develop different strategies to ensure that there is an infrastructure to deliver quality healthcare services in an organization.

■ Conclusion

Managers should be trained in human resource management concepts to be effective supervisors and leaders of their employees. This is true in small organizations that do not have the complex organizational structure to have a designated HR department. Most large organizations have a defined HR department that consists of both generalists and specialists in human resource functions that collaborate with managers to ensure they are managing their employees appropriately.

History indicates that human resource management activities were observed as early as 2000 B.C. Human resource management can be applied to any activity of a healthcare operation. It plays a role in the development of a legal and ethical workplace environment, provides information about healthcare careers to employees, assists with labor union negotiations, is responsible for job analysis and the hiring process, manages employee benefits, and provides input on employee performance. In addition, human resource management plays a role in emerging and future trends in health care and plays an integral role in strategic management including workforce planning.

■ Vocabulary

Accountable care organization
Allied health professionals
Efficiency
Employee benefits
Employee development

Employee training
Frederick W. Taylor
Global economy
Green House Project
Hawthorne studies

Health informatics
Health information systems
Health information technology
Human resource management
Industrial Revolution
Interprofessional education
Job analysis
Job design
Job enrichment
Job redesign
Job schedule redesign
Joint Commission
Labor unions
Legally defensible

Mandatory benefits
Medical informatics
Medical tourism
Occupational Safety and Health
   Administration
Pay for performance
Recruitment
Selection
Social media
Strategic planning
Team designs
U.S. Department of Labor
Value-based purchasing
Voluntary benefits

■ References

Accountable Care Organizations: Improving care coordination for people with Medicare. Available at: http://www.healthcare.gov/news/factsheets/2011/03/accountablecare03312011a.html. Accessed December 2, 2011.

Anderson, R., Rice, T. & Kominski, G. (2007). *Changing the U.S. Health Care System*. San Francisco, CA: Jossey-Bass.

Andrulis, D. (2003). Reducing racial and ethnic disparities in disease management to improve health outcomes. *Practical Disease Management*, 11(12):789–800.

Bureau of Labor Statistics (2011). Medical and health services managers. Available at: http://www.bls.gov/oco/ocos014.htm. Accessed December 2, 2011.

Byars, L. & Rue, L. (2006). *Human Resource Management* (eighth ed.). New York, NY: McGraw-Hill/Irwin, pp. 371–383.

Davis, C. (2010). Union membership grows among healthcare workers. Available at: http://www.fiercehealthcare.com/node/39662. Accessed October 30, 2010.

Department of Labor (2010). Chapter 1: Start Up of the Department. Available at: http://www.dol.gov/oasam/programs/history/dolchp01.htm. Accessed October 24, 2010.

Dessler, G. (2012). *Fundamentals of Human Resource Management*. Upper Saddle River, NJ: Prentice Hall, pp. 404–419.

Gentry, W. (2008). Health safety and preparedness. In Fried, B. & Fottler, M., eds. *Human Resources in Healthcare*. Chicago, IL: Health Administration Press, pp. 347–391.

Goldstein, M. & Blumenthal, D. (2008). Building an information technology infrastructure. *Journal of Law Medicine & Ethics*, 36(4):709–15.

High growth industry profile: Health care (2007). Available at: http://www.doleta.gov/BRG/Indprof/Healthcare_profile.cfm. Accessed December 2, 2011.

History of Human Resource Management (2010). Available at: http://buzzle.com/articles/history-of-human-resource-management.html. Accessed October 24, 2010.

Is the Latin American Health Insurance Market in Good Shape? (2011). Available at: http://www.globalsurance.com/blog/category/international-healthcare. Accessed December 2, 2011.

Kane, R., Lum, T., Cutler, L., Degenholtz, H. & Yu, T. (2007). Resident outcomes in small house nursing homes: A longitudinal evaluation of the initial Green House program. *Journal of Geriatrics Society*, 55(6):832–839.

Kinicki, A. & Willliams, B. (2008). *Management: A Practical Introduction* (3rd ed.). New York, NY: McGraw-Hill/Irwin, pp. 42–45.

Lewis, N. (2011). Most Health ITs Use Social Media. Available at: http://www.informationweek.com/news/healthcare/mobile-wireless/231601331. Accessed December 2, 2011.

Malvey, D. (2010). Unionization in healthcare: Background and trends. *Journal of Healthcare Management*, 55(3):154–157.

Mathis, R. & Jackson, J. (2006). *Human Resource Management* (11th ed.). Mason, OH: Thomson/Southwestern, pp. 524–565.

McKinnies, R., Collins, S., Collins, K. & Matthews, E. (2010). Lack of performance: The top reasons for terminating healthcare employees. *Journal of Radiology Management*, 32(3):44–47.

Minding the Workplace (2011). Available at: http://neworkplace.wordpress.com/2009/12/15/workplace-bullying-in-healthcare. Accessed June 10, 2011.

National Center for Health Statistics (2008). *Health, United States, 2008, with Chartbook*. Washington, DC: U.S. Government Printing Office. Available at: http://www.cdc.gov/nchs/data/hus/hus08.pdf. Accessed December 5, 2008.

Noe, R., Hollenbeck, J., Gerhart, B. & Wright, P. (20011). *Fundamentals of Human Resource Management* (4th ed.). New York, NY: McGraw-Hill/Irwin, pp. 30–31.

OSHA (2011). FAQ. Available at: http://www.osha.gov/OSHA_FAQs.html. Accessed June 2, 2011.

The Emergence of Modern Industrialism (2010). Available at: http://www.industrial-revolution.us. Accessed October 24, 2010.

Shi, L. & Singh, D. (2008). *An Introduction to Health Care in America: A Systems Approach*. Sudbury, MA: Jones and Bartlett Publishers.

Thompson, A., Strickland, A. & Gamble, J. (2010). *Crafting & Executing Strategy: The Quest for Competitive Advantage*. Boston, MA: McGraw-Hill/Irwin, pp. 1–15.

Zingheim, P. & Schuster, J. (2002). Creating a Workplace Business Brand. Available at: http://www.hr.com/hrcom. Accessed September 20, 2011.

STUDENT WORKBOOK ACTIVITY 1.1

Complete the following case scenarios based on the information provided in this chapter. Your answer must be *in your own words*.

Real-Life Applications: Case Scenario 1

Your friend knows that you are interested in becoming an HR manager for a healthcare organization. She has heard the term *human resources* many times but does not really understand how it developed as part of an organization.

Activity

You provide an early history of human resource management including the contributions of Frederick W. Taylor and the Hawthorne studies. Apply these contributions to the healthcare industry.

Responses

_____

_____

_____

_____

_____

_____

_____

_____

_____

_____

_____

_____

_____

_____

_____

_____

_____

_____

Real-Life Applications: Case Scenario 2

You understand that federal agencies often are responsible for monitoring and enforcing regulations in organizations.

Activity

You perform research to assess the roles of the Occupational Safety and Health Administration and the U.S. Department of Labor in monitoring the treatment of employees in healthcare organizations.

Responses

_____

_____

_____

_____

_____

_____

_____

_____

_____

_____

_____

_____

_____

_____

_____

_____

_____

Real-Life Applications: Case Scenario 3

You have decided that you are interested in human resource management as a career. You are not sure what types of HR activities are of interest to you.

Activity

To understand your choices, you list five HR activities that are used in a successful organization. Apply this to healthcare industries.

Responses

_____

_____

_____

_____

_____

_____

_____

_____

_____

_____

_____

_____

_____

_____

_____

Real-Life Applications: Case Scenario 4

Two trends affect how the healthcare industry operates.

Activity

Discuss the impact of the globalization of the economy and demographic and diversity trends on the healthcare industry.

Responses

_____

_____

_____

_____

_____

_____

_____

_____

_____

_____

_____

_____

_____

_____

_____

STUDENT WORKBOOK ACTIVITY 1.2

In Your Own Words

Based on this chapter, please provide an explanation of the following terms in your own words as they apply to human resource management. *Do not recite* the text.

Job analysis:

_____

_____

_____

Industrial Revolution:

_____

_____

_____

Employee training:

_____

_____

_____

Employee development:

_____

_____

_____

Health information technology:

_____

_____

_____

Job schedule redesign:

_____

_____

_____

Frederick W. Taylor:

_____

_____

_____

Hawthorne studies:

_____

_____

_____

Recruitment:

_____

_____

_____

Labor unions:

_____

_____

_____

STUDENT WORKBOOK ACTIVITY 1.3

Internet Exercises

Write your answers in the spaces provided.

- Visit each of the websites that are listed in the text that follows.
- Name the organization.
- Locate its mission statement on its website.

- Provide a brief overview of the activities of the organization.
- Apply this organization to the chapter information.

Websites

http://www.osha.gov

Organization name:

_____

Mission statement:

_____

_____

_____

Overview of activities:

_____

_____

_____

Application to chapter information:

_____

_____

_____

http://www.dol.gov

Organization name:

_____

Mission statement:

_____

_____

_____

Overview of activities:

_____

_____

_____

Application to chapter information:

_____

_____

_____

http://www.jointcommission.org
Organization name:

_____

Mission statement:

_____

_____

_____

Overview of activities:

_____

_____

_____

Application to chapter information:

_____

_____

_____

http://www.medicaltourism.com
Organization name:

_____

Mission statement:

_____

_____

_____

Overview of activities:

_____

_____

_____

Application to chapter information:

_____

_____

_____

http://www.shrm.org
Organization name:

_____

Mission statement:

_____

_____

_____

Overview of activities:

_____

_____

_____

Application to chapter information:

_____

_____

_____

http://www.fiercehealthcare.com

Organization name:

_____

Mission statement:

_____

_____

_____

Overview of activities:

_____

_____

_____

Application to chapter information:

_____

_____

_____

STUDENT ACTIVITY 1.4: DISCUSSION BOARDS FOR ONLINE, HYBRID, AND TRADITIONAL ONGROUND CLASSES
Discussion Board Guidelines

The discussion board is used in online and web-enhanced courses in place of classroom lectures and discussion. The board can also be used as an enhancement to traditional onground classes. The discussion board is the way in which the students "link together" as a class. The following are guidelines to help focus on the discussion topic and to define the roles and responsibilities of the discussion coordinator and other members of the class. The educator will be the discussion moderator for this course.

1. The educator will post the discussion topic and directions for the upcoming week. These postings should all be responses to the original topic or responses to other students' responses. When people respond to what someone else has posted, they should start the posting with the person's name so it is clear which message they are responding to. **A response such as "Yes" or "I agree" does not count for credit. Your responses must be in your own words. You cannot copy and paste from the text.**
2. Postings (especially responses) should include enough information so the message is clear but should not be so long that it becomes difficult to follow. Remember, this is like talking to someone in a classroom setting. The postings should reflect the content of the text or other assignments. If you retrieve information from the Internet, the hyperlink must be cited.
3. Students should check the discussion daily to see if new information has been posted that requires their attention and response.

Good discussion will often include different points of view. Students should feel free to disagree or "challenge" others to support their positions or ideas. All discussions must be handled in a respectful manner. The following are discussion boards for this chapter.

Discussion Boards

1. Define human resource management. Based on your experience, how do you think human resource management has played a role in your workplace?
2. Why is it important for employees to be familiar with legal and ethical issues in the healthcare workplace? Review Table 1.1. Which laws do you believe are the most important? Defend your answer.
3. What is the role of the Joint Commission in health care?
4. What is the importance of training employees? What type of training have you received as an employee? Was it successful? Have you ever trained another employee?

Be specific.

Legal, Ethical, and Safety Issues in the Healthcare Workplace

Learning Objectives

The student will be able to:

- Describe the legal relationship between patient and provider.
- Apply civil and criminal liability concepts to healthcare providers and consumers.
- Analyze six employment laws and their importance to the healthcare workplace.
- Examine the concept of ethics and its application to healthcare organizations.
- Discuss a healthcare ethical dilemma.

DID YOU KNOW THAT?

- The healthcare industry is one of the most regulated industries in the United States.
- The National Defense Authorization Act of 2008 allows an employee to take 12 weeks of unpaid leave if a child, spouse, or parent has been called to active duty.
- Voluntary hospitals are no longer exempt from lawsuits.
- According to civil law, surgery performed by a surgeon without consent could be considered assault and battery.
- Providers may order more tests and provide more services to protect themselves from medical malpractice lawsuits.

■ Introduction

To be an effective manager, it is important to understand basic legal and ethical principles that influence the work environment, including the legal relationship between the organization and the consumer—the healthcare provider and the patient. Ethical behavior, which is considered actions that are the right thing to do, not simply what is required by law, must also be described because the healthcare industry is fraught with difficult situations that involve ethical dilemmas. It is the responsibility of the human resources (HR) department to make employees knowledgeable in the information presented in this chapter. The basic concepts of law, both civil and criminal healthcare law, tort reform, employment-related legislation, safety in the workplace, workplace ethics, and the provider–patient relationship, healthcare organizational codes of ethics, public health ethics, research ethics, and workplace bullying will be described in this chapter.

■ Basic Concepts of Law in the Healthcare Workplace

The healthcare industry is one of the most heavily regulated industries in the United States. Those who provide, receive, pay for, and regulate healthcare services are affected by the law (Miller, 2006a). **Law** is a body of rules for the conduct of individuals and organizations. Law is created so that there is a minimal standard of action required by individuals and organizations. There exist laws created by federal, state, and local governments. When the judiciary system interprets previous legal decisions with respect to a case, they create **common law** (Buchbinder & Shanks, 2007). The minimal standard for action is federal law, although state law may be more stringent. Legislatures create laws that are called **statutes**. Both common law and statutes are then interpreted by administrative agencies by developing **rules and regulations** that interpret the law.

There exist civil and criminal laws that affect the healthcare industry. **Civil law** focuses on the wrongful acts against individuals and organizations based on contractual violations. In civil law, **torts**, derived from the French word for *wrong*, is a category of wrongful acts or negligence that can result in different types of healthcare violations. To prove a civil infraction, you do not need as much evidence as in a criminal case. **Criminal law** is concerned with actions that are illegal based on court decisions. To convict someone of a criminal activity, it has to be proved without a reasonable doubt of guilt. Examples of criminal law infractions would be Medicare and Medicaid fraud (Miller, 2006b).

As stated earlier, torts are wrongdoings that occur to individuals or organizations regardless of whether a contract is in place. Medical malpractice cases are examples of torts. There are several different types of violations that can apply to health care. There are two basic healthcare torts: (1) **negligence**, which involves the unintentional act or omission of an act that could negatively contribute to the health of a patient, and (2) **intentional torts**, such as assault and battery and invasion of privacy (Buchbinder & Shanks, 2007).

An example of negligence is if a provider does not give appropriate care or withholds care that results in damages to the patient's health. In the healthcare industry, intentional torts such as **assault** and **battery** would be a surgeon performing surgery on a patient without his or her consent (Miller, 2006c). An example of **invasion of privacy** would be the violation of patients' health records. Privacy relating to patient information is a major issue in the healthcare industry. As more information that is confidential is shared electronically, there is an increased risk of invasion of privacy. These examples are categorized under the term *medical malpractice*.

According to the *American Heritage Dictionary*, **medical malpractice** is the "Improper or negligent treatment of a patient by a provider which results in injury, damage or loss" (*American Heritage Dictionary*, 2000). According to the Institute of Medicine's landmark report *To Err Is Human*, medical malpractice results in approximately 80,000 to 100,000 deaths per year. The Congressional Budget Office (CBO) found that in 2003 there were over 180,000 severe injuries due to medical negligence. Harvard School of Medicine researchers indicate that in 2005 nearly 20% of hospital patients are injured during their care (Medical Negligence, 2011). Disputes over improper care of a patient have hurt both providers and patients. Patients have sued physicians because of the belief that the physician has not given the patient a level of care comparable with the **standard of care** established in the industry.

■ Tort Reform Discussion

As a result of the number of malpractice claims in the United States, malpractice insurance premiums have increased, which has resulted in the introduction of **defensive medicine**, which means that providers order more tests and provide more services than necessary to protect themselves from malpractice lawsuits (Shi & Singh, 2008a). In addition, some states are no longer offering malpractice insurance, which means there are fewer physicians in needed areas resulting in geographic maldistribution of physicians. Malpractice insurance crises occurred during the 1970s and 1980s (Danzon, 1995). The issues in the 1970s led to joint underwriting measures that required insurance companies to offer medical malpractice if the physician purchased other insurance. In some states, compensation funds were established to offset large award settlements. The number of malpractice suits decreased, but the amounts of awards were still huge. During the mid-1980s, the premiums rose again—nearly 75% (Rosenbach & Stone, 1990). A third malpractice insurance crisis occurred in the first decade of the 21st century. Issues with obtaining medical malpractice insurance in several states have increased, forcing physicians to turn to joint underwriting associations, which can charge exorbitant premiums.

As a result of the recent malpractice insurance crisis, more states have adopted statutory caps on monetary damages that a plaintiff can recover in malpractice claims. States believe that a **monetary cap** on malpractice claims would limit the increase of malpractice insurance premiums. The less an insurance company has paid out in malpractice insurance claims, the less the insurance company would have to raise insurance rates. According to the National Conference of State Legislatures, in 2005 there were 48 states that considered malpractice reform legislation with 30 states adopting law (Waters, Budetti, Claxton & Lundy, 2007). For example, Nevada adopted a cap of $350,000 on noneconomic damages in medical malpractice cases. However, some state appellate courts have declared caps to be unconstitutional (Nelson, Morrisey & Kilgore, 2007). Studies have been contradictory regarding the positive impact that monetary caps have on reducing malpractice insurance rates. States have also developed several other **tort reform** measures that relate to filing claims such as limiting attorney's fees, setting a statute of limitations on claims, and adhering to alternative dispute resolution methods, which are typically less costly than court disputes.

Many legal factors have also contributed to the increase in claims. **Voluntary hospitals,** which are private and not for profit, are no longer exempt from malpractice suits. Employers now have to take responsibility for their employees' wrongdoing. The concept of **informed consent** parameters, which means the patient is provided accurate information prior to any medical treatment, has expanded and therefore increased claims have occurred. The acceptable **standard of care,** which used to be strictly based on a similar community's medical care standard, has now become a state or national standard, which has also resulted in increased claims (Miller, 2006c).

Expert witness qualifications are also specified to ensure that the witness is an expert in his or her field. Clinical practice guidelines, which are developed to ensure an acceptable standard of care, are also used (Miller, 2006d). The informed consent of a patient to receive care was also expanded in the 1970s to become a patient-friendly standard that specifies what information must be given to the patient to ensure he or she is making an informed decision regarding his or her care (Office of Technology Assessment, 1993).

Some physicians are leaving private practice because they can no longer afford the premiums—they are now in administrative positions at all levels of government, are academicians, or teach at medical universities. The malpractice insurance issues have forced many states to review their malpractice guidelines. In some states, tort reform that has imposed limits on the amount awarded continues to cause controversy. However, recent federal studies have indicated that imposing caps on awards may be an effective method to reduce malpractice costs and to discourage frivolous lawsuits. In addition, the U.S. Supreme Court ruled that any awards must be included in an individual's taxed income (Miller, 2006e).

It is the responsibility of the HR department to ensure that healthcare employees are aware of these litigious issues and are trained to deal with patients in accordance with these legal issues. HR management must also train employees with respect to the impact of employment-related healthcare legislation. The following section outlines major human resources-related legislation that influences the healthcare industry (Table 2.1).

■ Human Resource-Related Legislation

Equal Pay Act of 1963 (Amended FLSA)

This act, which amended the Fair Labor Standards Act and is enforced by the U.S. Department of Labor, mandates that all employers award pay fairly to both genders

Table 2.1 Major Human Resource-Related Legislation

Equal Pay Act of 1963: All employers must provide equal pay to both genders that have the same position with equal responsibilities and skills. Enforced by the U.S. Department of Labor.

Civil Rights Act of 1964, Title VII: Landmark legislation. Prohibits discrimination of protected classes based on gender, race, color, religion, and national origin. Enforced by the EEOC. Applies to employers with 15 or more employees.

Age Discrimination in Employment Act of 1967 (ADEA): Protects employees and job applicants 40 years or older from discrimination in hiring, firing, promotion, layoffs, training, benefits, and assignments. Enforced by EEOC. Applies to employers with 20 or more employees.

Occupational Safety and Health Act of 1970: This act requires employers to provide a safe and healthy work environment. Guidelines for working with hazardous chemicals and for working ergonomically. Enforced by the Occupational Safety and Health Administration.

Rehabilitation Act of 1973: Employers with 50 or more employees and with federal funding of $50,000 must submit an affirmative action plan. Amended to ensure that healthcare facilities are accessible for the disabled. Enforced by the Office of Federal Contract Compliance Programs.

Employee Retirement Income Security Act of 1974 (ERISA): Regulates pensions and benefit plans for employees. Forbids employers from firing employees so the employers do not have to pay the employee's medical coverage. Gives employees the right to sue for breaches of any fiduciary duty. Enforced by the U.S. Department of Labor.

Pregnancy Discrimination Act of 1978: Protects female employees who are pregnant against discrimination. Applied to employers with 15 or more employees. Enforced by the EEOC.

Consolidated Omnibus Budget Reconciliation Act of 1986 (COBRA): Passed to ensure that if an individual changes jobs, he or she can still obtain health insurance. Enforced by the U.S. Department of Labor.

Worker Adjustment and Retraining Notification Act of 1989: Employers with 100 employees or more must give their employees 60 days notice of layoffs and closings. U.S. Department of Labor has no enforcement role but can assist with job placement.

Americans with Disabilities Act of 1990 (ADA): Protects the disabled from employment discrimination. Encourages businesses to provide reasonable accommodation in the workplace for qualified individuals that have disabilities but are able to perform a job. Applies to employers with 15 or more employees. Enforced by the EEOC. Its 2008 amendments expanded the concept of disabilities.

(continues)

Table 2.1 (Continued)

Older Workers Benefit Protection Act of 1990 (OWBA): Amended the ADEA. Benefits must be provided to both younger and older workers. Gives time to accept early retirement options and allows employees to change their mind if they want to litigate against their company. Enforced by the EEOC.

Civil Rights Act of 1991: Amendment to 1964 Act. Enables individuals to receive monetary damages up to $300,000 because of intentional discrimination. Enforced by the EEOC. Applies to employers with 15 or more employees. This Act also established the Glass Ceiling Commission that examined the lack of protected classes in senior management positions.

Family Medical Leave Act of 1993 (FMLA): Requires employers with 50 or more employees within a 75-mile radius who work more than 25 hours per week and who have been employed more than 1 year to provide up to 12 work weeks of unpaid leave to an employee during any 12-month period so the employee may provide care for a family member or obtain care for himself or herself. Enforced by the U.S. Department of Labor.

Uniformed Services Employment and Reemployment Rights Act of 1994 (USERRA): Workers are entitled to return to their job after military service. Returning employees are not penalized from raises or promotions because they were in the military. The U.S. Department of Labor's (DOL) Veterans' Employment and Training Service (VETS) enforces USERRA.

Health Insurance Portability and Accountability Act of 1996 (HIPAA): Increased restrictions on patient information confidentiality by creating a standard for patient information sharing. Enforced by U.S. Health and Human Services.

Pension Protection Act of 2006: Amendment to Civil Rights Act of 1991. Landmark legislation that strengthens employer funding requirements for employee pension plans and creates a stronger pension insurance system. Enforced by the U.S. Department of Labor.

National Defense Authorization Act of 2008: Expanded the FMLA to include families of military service members, which means that an employee may take up to 12 weeks of leave if a child, spouse, or parent has been called to active duty in the armed forces. Enforced by the U.S. Department of Labor.

Genetic Information Nondiscrimination Act of 2008: Prohibits U.S. insurance companies and employers from discriminating based on genetic test results. Enforced by the EEOC.

Table 2.1 (Continued)

Lilly Ledbetter Fair Pay Act of 2009: An amendment to Title VII of the Civil Rights Act of 1964 that also applies to claims under the Age Discrimination in Employment Act of 1967 and ADA and provides protection for unlawful employment practices related to compensation discrimination. Enforced by the EEOC.

Patient Protection and Affordable Care Act of 2010 (PPACA): Controversial legislation that requires individuals to purchase health insurance by 2014. Contested by several states for its constitutionality, provisions of the Act will be reviewed by the Supreme Court in 2012.

if it is determined their jobs have equal responsibilities and require the same skills. It can be difficult to assess whether two employees are performing the exact same job. One employee may have additional duties, which would affect his or her pay. The current trend in business is pay for performance, so some employees may earn more if they perform better. However, research consistently states that women earn less than men do. An individual who alleges pay discrimination may file a lawsuit without informing the EEOC.

Civil Rights Act of 1964, Title VII

This landmark act prohibits discrimination based on race, sex, color, religion, and national origin. Discrimination means making distinctions among people that are different. This legislation is the key legal piece to equal opportunity employment. Two components to this legislation, which will be discussed later, are disparate treatment and disparate impact. This legislation applies to employers with 15 or more employees. The act is enforced by the Equal Employment Opportunity Commission (EEOC).

The Civil Rights Act of 1964, Title VII, created a concept of protected classes to protect these groups from employment discrimination of compensation, conditions, or privileges of employment. The protected classes include sex, age, national origin, race, and religion. A major current issue under the purview of discrimination legislation is sexual harassment. According to the EEOC, **sexual harassment** is defined as unwelcome sexual conduct that has a negative impact on the employee. There are two major distinctions in sexual harassment: (1) quid pro quo sexual harassment, which occurs when sexual activities occur in return for an employment benefit, and (2) when the behavior of coworkers is sexual in nature and creates an uncomfortable work environment. What is more prevalent in sexual harassment is the creation of a hostile work environment. Several court case judgments indicate that repeated suggestive joke telling or lewd photos on display can be legally constituted as a hostile work environment. In the healthcare industry, nurses experience sexual harassment from colleagues, physicians, and patients.

Age Discrimination in Employment Act of 1967

This act protects employees and job applicants 40 years and older from discrimination as it applies to hiring, firing, promotion, layoffs, training, assignments, and benefits. Older employees file lawsuits for age discrimination in job termination. This legislation applies to employers with 20 or more employees and the act is enforced by the EEOC. During difficult economic times, older employees' complaints of termination increase.

Consumer Credit Protection Act (Title III) of 1968

This act prohibits employers from terminating an employee if the individual's earnings are subject to garnishment due to debt issues. This Act also limits the weekly garnishment amount from the individual's pay. The Act is enforced by the Federal Deposit Insurance Corporation.

Occupational Safety and Health Act of 1970

The OSHA Act of 1970 requires employers to provide a safe and healthy place of employment. It established the Occupational Safety and Health Administration, which collaborates with states on policies for safe work environments.

Rehabilitation Act of 1973

This law applies to organizations that receive financial assistance from federal organizations, including the U.S. Department of Health and Human Services, to prevent discrimination against individuals with disabilities with respect to receipt of employee benefits and job opportunities. These organizations and employers include many hospitals, nursing homes, mental health centers, and human service programs. Employers with 50 or more employees and federal contracts of $50,000 or more must submit written affirmative action plans. The act is enforced by the Office of Federal Contract Compliance Programs (OFCCP).

Employee Retirement Income Security Act of 1974

The Employee Retirement Income Security Act of 1974 (ERISA) regulates pension and benefit plans for employees, including medical and disability benefits. It protects employees because it forbids employers from firing an employee so that the employee cannot collect under their medical coverage. An employee may change the benefits provided under his or her plan, but employers cannot force an employee to leave so that the employer does not have to pay the employee's medical coverage.

Pregnancy Discrimination Act of 1978 (Amendment to CRA 1964)

This is an amendment to Title VII of the Civil Rights Act of 1964. This act protects female employees that are discriminated against based on pregnancy-related conditions, which constitutes illegal sex discrimination. A pregnant woman must be treated like anyone with a medical condition. For example, an organization must allow sick leave for pregnant women with morning sickness if they also allow sick leave for other nausea illnesses (Gomez-Mejia et al., 2012). This legislation applies to employers with 15 or more employees and is enforced by the EEOC.

Consolidated Omnibus Budget Reconciliation Act of 1986

The Consolidated Omnibus Budget Reconciliation Act of 1986 (COBRA), an amendment to ERISA, was passed to protect employees who lost or changed employers so that they could keep their health insurance if they paid 102% of the full premium (Anderson, Rice & Kominski, 2007b). The act was passed because, at the time, people were afraid to change jobs, resulting in the concept of **job lock** (Emanuel, 2008). COBRA also includes provisions that require hospitals to provide care to everyone who presented at an emergency department, regardless of their ability to pay. Fines were accrued if it was determined that hospitals were refusing treatment (Sultz & Young, 2006). This component was very important because many individuals were refused treatment because they could not pay for the services or were uninsured.

Immigration Reform and Control Act of 1988

The Immigration Reform and Control Act of 1988 requires employers with one or more employees to verify that all job applicants are U.S. citizens or authorized to work in the United States. Most employees are only aware of this legislation because of the I-9 form all new employees must complete. There are three categories, A, B, and C, on the form. Category A establishes identity and eligibility to work such as by a passport, Permanent Resident Card, or Permanent Alien Registration Receipt Card. Category B establishes identity of the individual. Acceptable proof of identify includes a driver's license and different types of identification cards with photographs. Category C focuses on eligibility of an employee to work. Documentation includes a Social Security card or birth certificate. If an employee cannot provide this information, he or she must provide documentation in both Category B and Category C. This prohibits any company from hiring illegal aliens and penalizes employers who hire illegal aliens. However, immigrants with special skill sets or who can satisfy a labor shortage in the United States, such as nurses, will be permitted to work in the United States. This act is enforced by the U.S. Department of Labor.

Drug Free Workplace Act of 1988

This act requires any employers who receive federal grants or who have a federal contract of $25,000 or greater to certify that they operate a drug-free workplace. They must provide education to their employees about drug abuse. Many employers now offer drug testing. This act is enforced by the U.S. Department of Labor.

Worker Adjustment and Retraining Notification Act of 1989

Employers who have 100 employees or more must give their employees 60 days notice of layoffs and business closings. This act is enforced by the U.S. Department of Labor.

Americans with Disabilities Act of 1990

The Americans with Disabilities Act of 1990 (ADA) focuses on individuals who are considered disabled in the workplace. There are three sections: Section I contains employment limitations, and Section II and Section III target local government organizations, hotels, restaurants, and grocery stores. This legislation applies to employers who have 15 employees or more and is enforced by the EEOC. According to the law, a disabled person is someone who has a physical or mental impairment that limits the ability to hear, see, speak, or walk. The act was passed to ensure that those individuals who had a disability but who could perform primary job functions were not discriminated against. According to the act, the disabilities include learning disabilities, mental disabilities, epilepsy, cancer, arthritis, mental retardation, AIDS, asthma, and traumatic brain injury. A nursing home cannot refuse to admit a person with AIDS that requires a nursing service if the hospital has that type of service available (Americans with Disabilities Act of 1990, 2011). Alcohol and other drug abuses are not covered under ADA. Individuals who are morbidly obese can be considered disabled if the obesity was related to a physical cause.

Title I of ADA states that employment discrimination is prohibited against individuals with disabilities who can perform **essential functions** of a job with or without *reasonable* accommodation. Essential functions are job duties that must be performed for an individual to be a satisfactory employee. Reasonable accommodation refers to employers that take reasonable action to accommodate a disabled individual such as providing special computer equipment or furniture to accommodate a physical limitation. The reasonable accommodation should not cause undue financial hardship to the employer.

Individuals with disabilities have mental or physical limitations such as walking, speaking, breathing, sitting, seeing, or hearing. **Intellectual disabilities** refer to an IQ less than 70–75, the disability occurred before 18 years of age, and the individual has issues with social skills. Intellectual disabilities must significantly limit major life activities such as walking, seeing, hearing, thinking, speaking, learning, concentrating, and working. The ADA amendments of 2008 expanded living activities to include bodily functions such as bladder, circulatory, neurologic, and digestive functions.

Older Workers Benefit Protection Act of 1990 (Amendment to ADEA)

This act amended the Age Discrimination in Employment Act. Its goal was to ensure that older workers' employee benefits were protected and that an organization provided the same benefits to both younger and older workers. The act also gives employees time to decide if they would accept early retirement options and allows employees to change their mind if they have signed a waiver for their right to sue. This act is enforced by the EEOC.

Civil Rights Act of 1991 (Amendment to CRA of 1964)

Title VII only allowed damages for back pay. This act enables individuals to receive both **punitive damages**, which are damages that punish the defendant, and **compensatory damages** for financial or psychological harm. This legislation applies to employers with 15 or more employees. The size of the damages is based on the size of the company: $50,000 for employers with 15 to 100 employees; $100, 000 for employers with 101 to 200 employees; $200,000 for employers with 201 to 500 employees; and $300,000 for employers with more than 500 employees. This act is enforced by the EEOC.

The 1991 law extended the possibility of individuals collecting damages related to sex, religious, or disability-related discrimination. Organizations had developed a policy of adjusting scores on employment tests so that a certain percentage of a protected class would be hired. This amendment to Title VII specifically prohibits quotas, which are diversity goals to increase the number of a protected class in a workforce (Gomez-Mejia, Balkin & Cardy, 2012). The amendment also created the Glass Ceiling Commission, which examined the lack of protected classes in senior management positions (1991–1996).

Family Medical Leave Act of 1993

The Family Medical Leave Act of 1993 (FMLA) requires employers with 50 or more employees within a 75-mile radius who work more than 25 hours per week and who have been employed more than 1 year to provide up to 12 work weeks of unpaid leave to an employee during any 12-month period so the employee may provide care for a family member or obtain care for himself or herself. This benefit can also include post-childbirth or adoption. The employer must provide healthcare benefits although it is not required to provide wages. This benefit does not cover the organization's 10% highest paid employees. The employer is also supposed to provide the same job or a comparable position upon the return of the employee (Noe, Hollenbeck, Gerhart & Wright, 2009).

Health Insurance Portability and Affordability Act of 1996

The Health Insurance Portability and Affordability Act of 1996 (HIPAA) was passed to promote patient information and confidentiality in a secure environment. Fully implemented in 2003, the amount of health information released is controlled by the consumer. This is the first federal legislation that provides in-depth protection of consumers' health information. Both civil and criminal penalties, including incarceration, were included in this act. Civil penalties were capped at $100 per violation and $25,000 per year. Criminal penalties ranged from $50,000 to $250,000 with 1–10 years of incarceration (Stanwyck & Stanwyck, 2009).

HIPAA was an amendment to ERISA and the Public Health Service Act to increase access to healthcare coverage when employees changed jobs. HIPAA made it illegal to obtain personal medical information for reasons other than healthcare activities, which also includes genetic information. It also guaranteed that individuals could purchase health insurance for a preexisting condition if they (1) have been covered by a previous employer program for a minimum of 18 months, (2) have exhausted any coverage through COBRA, (3) are ineligible for other health insurance programs, and (4) were uninsured for no longer than 2 months. Other provisions include (1) small businesses with 2–50 employees cannot be refused insurance, (2) self-employed individuals are allowed an increased tax deduction (30% to 80% by 2006) for health insurance premiums, and (3) employers or insurance companies cannot drop individuals for high usage of their medical plans (Shi & Singh, 2008b). This act is enforced by the U.S. Department of Health and Human Services Office for Civil Rights and by the U.S. Department of Justice.

Mental Health Parity Act of 1996

This act defines the equality or parity between lifetime and annual limits of health insurance reimbursements on both mental health and medical care. Unfortunately, the act did not require employers to offer mental health coverage, it did not impose limits on deductibles or coinsurance payments, nor did it cover substance abuse. This federal legislation spurred several states to implement their own parity legislation (Anderson, Rice & Kominski, 2007b).

HIPAA National Standards to Protect Patients' Personal Medical Records of 2002

This legislation amended the HIPAA, further protecting medical records and other personal health information maintained by healthcare providers, hospitals, insurance companies, and health plans. It gives patients new rights to access of their records, restricts the amount of patient information released, and establishes new restrictions to researchers' access (The Privacy Rule, 2011).

The Wellstone Act, or the Mental Health Parity and Addiction Equity Act of 2008, amends the Mental Health Parity Act of 1996 to include substance abuse treatment plans as part of group health plans.

National Defense Authorization Act of 2008

This act expanded FMLA to include families of military service members, which means that an employee may take up to 12 weeks of leave if a child, spouse, or parent has been called to active duty in the armed forces. Additionally, if a service member is injured or ill as a result of active duty, the employee may take up to 26 weeks of leave in a single 12-month leave year (Hickman, Gilligan & Patton, 2008).

Genetic Information Nondiscrimination Act of 2008

This act prohibits U.S. insurance companies and employers from discriminating based on information derived from genetic tests. Specifically, it forbids insurance companies from discriminating through reduced coverage or price increases. It also prohibits employers from making adverse employment decisions based on a person's genetic code. Employers or insurance companies cannot demand a genetic test (National Human Genome Research Institute, 2009).

Health Information Technology for Economic and Clinical Health Act of 2009

Effective September 23, 2009, this act amends HIPAA by requiring stricter notification protocols for breach of any patient information. These new rules apply to any associates of the health plans. It also increased HIPAA's civil and criminal penalties for violating consumer privacy regarding personal health information. Civil penalties were increased to $1,500,000 per calendar year, which was a huge increase in the original penalty cap of $25,000. The criminal penalties of up to $50,000 to $250,000 and 10 years of incarceration remained the same.

Lilly Ledbetter Fair Pay Act of 2009

This act, an amendment to Title VII of the Civil Rights Act of 1964 that also applies to claims under the Age Discrimination in Employment Act of 1967 and the Americans with Disabilities Act of 1990, provides protection for unlawful employment practices related to compensation discrimination. This act was named after Lilly Ledbetter, an employee of Goodyear Tire and Rubber Company who found out near her retirement that her male colleagues were paid more than she was. The U.S. Supreme Court ruled that she should have filed a suit within 180 days of the date that Goodyear paid her less than her peers. This act allows the statute of limitations to restart every 180 days from the time the worker receives a paycheck (Drachsler, 2010).

To avoid litigation, Sedhom (2009) suggests the implementation of a program coordinated by senior management and HR to help protect employers from being accused of unfair employment practices. The following summarizes the steps of the program:

1. Establish compensation criteria.
2. Develop pay audits and document these audits for several years.
3. Document retention processes related to pay.

4. Train managers on providing objective performance evaluations.
5. Develop and implement a rigorous statistical analysis of pay distributions.

Patient Protection and Affordability Care Act of 2010

This healthcare legislation has been controversial. There were national public protests and a huge division among the political parties regarding the components of the legislation. People, in general, agreed that the U.S. healthcare system needed some type of reform, but it was difficult to develop common recommendations that had majority support. Criticism, in part, focused on the increased role of government in monitoring the healthcare system and requiring individuals to obtain health insurance.

The one implementation that has been generally supported is the expansion of the dependent coverage provided by parental health insurance from age 25 until age 26, even if the child is not living with his or her parents, is not declared a dependent on the parents' tax return, is a student, or is no longer a student. This would not apply to individuals who have employer-based coverage (Kolpack, 2010). Another positive mandate, implemented in July 2010, was the establishment of a web portal, www.healthcare.gov, to increase consumer awareness about eligibility for specific healthcare insurance.

In addition to the two reforms discussed in the previous paragraphs, the following are selected major reforms that were also implemented in 2010:

- Elimination of lifetime and annual caps on healthcare reimbursement.
- Provision of assistance for the uninsured with preexisting conditions.
- Creation of a temporary reinsurance program for early retirees.

In the past, health insurance companies would establish an annual or lifetime cap of reimbursement for the use of healthcare insurance. These would be eliminated. Unlike the past, health insurance companies would also be prohibited from dropping individuals and children with certain conditions or not providing insurance to those individuals with preexisting conditions. The government would provide assistance to securing healthcare insurance for these high-risk individuals.

The following are selected major reforms that will be implemented by 2014:

- Insurance companies will be prohibited from setting insurance rates based on health status, medical condition, genetic information, or other related factors.
- Each state must establish the American Health Benefit Exchange, which is a marketplace where consumers can obtain information and buy health insurance.
- Most individuals must maintain minimum essential healthcare coverage or pay a fine of $95, $350 in 2015, $750 in 2016, and indexed after that year.
- Employers who have 200 or more employees must automatically enroll new full-time employees in healthcare coverage. Employers will also receive tax credits depending on their size.

In the past, there were issues with health insurance companies denying coverage based on health status or other conditions. Premiums now will be based on family type, geography, tobacco use, and age. In addition, each state will establish an American Health Benefit Exchange to assist consumers with obtaining health insurance. Funding is available to states to establish the exchanges within 1 year of enactment of the law, up to January 1, 2015. There will be Public Plan Options and Consumer Operated and Oriented Plans. The Public Plan Option will be a federal contract with insurers to offer two multi-state plans in each exchange of which one plan must be offered by a nonprofit organization. The Consumer Operated and Oriented Plans are member-run health organizations in all 50 states and must be consumer focused with profits targeted to lowering premiums and improving benefits.

The Small Business Option Program will allow small businesses to purchase coverage starting in 2017. The information will be provided to consumers in a standardized format so they can compare the plans. Plans and cost will vary based on level of coverage. There are exceptions based on circumstances. Employers with 200 employees or more must also enroll new employees in a healthcare plan. The purpose of these programs is to increase the number of consumers who have access to affordable health care. By 2014, most consumers will be responsible for obtaining healthcare insurance or pay a fine as described earlier. The PPACA has affected how health insurance companies provide coverage (Niles, 2010).

Role of the Equal Employment Opportunity Commission

The EEOC was created by Title VII of the Civil Rights Act of 1964. It is responsible for processing complaints, issuing regulations, and collecting information from employers. The EEOC collaborates with other federal agencies such as the U.S. Department of Labor to ensure that employees are treated fairly.

Processing Complaints

If an individual feels discriminated against, he or she files a complaint with the EEOC, which, in turn, notifies the employer. The employer is responsible for safeguarding any written information regarding the complaint. The EEOC then investigates the complaint to determine if the employer did violate any laws. If a violation was found, the EEOC uses conciliation or negotiation to resolve the issue without going to court. If conciliation is not successful, litigation or going to trial is the next step. Most employers prefer to avoid litigation because it is costly and damages their reputation. Most cases are resolved by conciliation.

Issuing Regulations

The EEOC is responsible for developing regulations for any EEOC laws and their amendments. They have written regulations and amendments for the ADA, ADEA, and Equal Pay Act. They also issue guidelines for different issues such as sexual harassment and affirmative action.

An **affirmative action plan** is a strategy that encourages employers to increase the diversity of their workforces by hiring individuals based on race, sex, and age. These potential employees must be qualified for the job. Although an affirmative action plan encourages hiring protected class candidates, an employer cannot set quotas for this process. They can develop strategies to encourage applications by diverse candidates.

An employer who develops an affirmative action plan must perform an analysis of the demographics of the current workforce compared with the eligible pool of qualified applicants. The employer must also calculate the percentage of the protected class among the qualified applicants. The percentages are compared to determine if there is an underrepresentation of diverse employees in the organization. If it is determined that the current workforce is not diverse, then an employer develops a timetable to hire diverse employees, which also includes a recruitment plan.

Information and Education

The EEOC acquires information from employers regarding their practices. Employers with 100 or more employees must file an EEO-1 report, which reflects the number of women and minorities who hold positions. This report is used to assess any potential discrimination trends. The EEOC also provides written and electronic media education about discrimination to employers. They send this information to the HR departments, which disseminate the information with training classes.

These pieces of legislation focus on equal employment opportunity in the workplace. These laws ensure that protected classes, as outlined in the Civil Rights Act of 1964, are provided opportunities for equal employment without bias or discrimination. In addition to this landmark legislation, the Age in Discrimination Act, Older Workers Benefit Protection Act, and the ADA establish standards for treating individuals who are older than 40 years, and those individuals who have a disability are also treated fairly in their terms of employment. Both the Age in Discrimination Act and the ADA were further strengthened by the passage of the Lilly Ledbetter Fair Pay Act regarding pay discrimination. In addition, the Pregnancy Discrimination Act and the Equal Pay Act target discrimination against women. Despite the number of antidiscrimination pieces of legislation, discrimination continues to exist in the work environment.

The release of patient information is more complex because of the introduction of information technology to the healthcare industry. For example, patient information may be faxed as long as only necessary information is transmitted and safeguards are implemented. Physicians may also communicate via e-mail as long as safeguards are implemented.

Role of the Occupational Safety and Health Administration

Part of the U.S. Department of Labor, this federal agency is very important to the healthcare industry because of the high incidence of employee injury. It enforces the regulations of the OSHA of 1970. There is a high risk of exposure to workplace hazards such as airborne and blood-borne infectious diseases, physical injuries from the lifting of patients, and needle-stick injuries. This law was passed to ensure that employers have a **general duty** to provide a safe and healthy work environment for their employees, which is very important for the healthcare industry because of potential exposure to bacteria, viruses, and contaminated fluids. Employers are also required to inform employees of potential hazardous conditions and Occupational Safety and Health Administration (OSHA) standards. Posters and other materials are posted for the education of employees. OSHA is responsible for enforcing these provisions. The National Institute for Occupational Safety and Health (NIOSH) was also established as part of this act to provide research to support the standards. OSHA enforces the **Hazard Communication standard,** which requires companies to label hazardous materials. Information is contained in **Material Safety Data Sheets** (MSDSs), which are provided to employees via the Internet or on site. OSHA has also issued a standard for exposure to human immunodeficiency virus, hepatitis B virus, and other blood-borne pathogens. This standard is crucial to the healthcare industry because of increased risk of exposure by nurses and laboratory workers.

OSHA has also developed standards for **personal protective equipment,** which mandate equipment to be used in situations of personal exposure to hazardous materials or working conditions. Companies must also maintain records of employee accidents. OSHA provides workers with the rights to receive training, to keep a copy of their medical records, and to request OSHA inspections of their workplace.

OSHA has also developed standards for **ergonomics,** which is the study of working conditions that affect the physical condition of employees. Studies indicate that repetitive motion can create employee injuries. A common disorder is **carpal tunnel syndrome,** which is a wrist injury common to repetitive hand motion that occurs in jobs such as that of grocery cashier and in computer users. Employers can provide ergonomic-friendly equipment and guidelines for ergonomic actions to eliminate these types of injuries. Ergonomic equipment and actions are important to the healthcare industry because many workers often lift patients to and from beds, operating tables, and wheelchairs (OSHA, 2010).

■ Basic Concepts of Ethics in the Healthcare Workplace

Ethical standards are considered one level above legal standards because individuals make a choice based on what is the "right thing to do," or what one ought to do, not what are the minimal actions required by law. There are many interpretations of the concept of ethics. Ethics has been interpreted as the moral foundation for standards of conduct (Taylor, 1975). The concept of **ethical standards** applies to actions that are hoped for and expected by individuals. There are many definitions of ethics but, basically, **ethics** is concerned with what are right and wrong choices as perceived by society and its individuals. Ethical dilemmas are often a conflict between personal and professional ethics. A **healthcare ethical dilemma** is a problem, situation, or opportunity that requires an individual, such as a healthcare provider, to choose an action between two obligations (Niles, 2010). The dilemma occurs when the ethical reasoning of the decision maker may conflict with the ethical reasoning of the patient and the institution. Dilemmas are often resolved because of the guidelines provided by codes of ethics of medical associations or healthcare institutions, ethics training, and implementation of ethical decision-making models.

According to Beauchamp and Childress (2001) and Gillon (1994), the role of ethics in the healthcare industry is based on five basic values that all healthcare providers should observe:

- **Respect for autonomy**: Decision making may be different, and healthcare providers must respect their patients' decisions.
- **Beneficence**: The healthcare provider should have the patient's best interests in mind.
- **No malfeasance**: The healthcare provider will not cause any harm when taking action.
- **Justice**: Healthcare providers will make fair decisions.
- **Dignity**: Patients should be treated with respect and dignity.

Autonomy, which is defined as self-rule, is an important concept to health care because it is applied to informed consent, which requires a provider to obtain the approval of a patient who has been provided adequate information to make a decision regarding intervention. Informed consent is a legal requirement for medical intervention. As part of the autonomy concept, it is also important that the provider respect the decision of the patient even if the patient's decisions do not agree with the provider's recommendation. A friend who has been diagnosed with a very advanced stage of cancer was told by her provider that she could enroll her in an experimental program that would give her 2 to 3 months to live. The intervention is very potent with severe side effects. My friend decided to try a homeopathic medicine to attack her disease. Her doctor was not in agreement with her choice, but she respected her patient's decision. She told her that if she needed pain medication, she could come and see her, and she would help her. This situation is an excellent example of autonomy in medicine.

Beneficence means that the best interest of the patient should always be the first priority of the healthcare provider, and **no malfeasance** states that healthcare providers must not take any actions to harm the patient. As discussed in the paragraph on autonomy, the concepts of beneficence and no malfeasance appear to be very easy to understand; however, there may be a difference of interpretation between the provider and the patient as to what is best for the patient. For example, Jehovah's Witnesses, a religious sect, do not believe in blood transfusions and will not give consent during an operation for a transfusion to occur, despite the procedure's ability to possibly save a life (Miller, 2006f). The provider has been trained to believe in beneficence and no malfeasance. However, from the provider's point of view, if the provider respects the wishes of the patient and family, he or she will potentially be harming the patient.

Justice or fairness in health care emphasizes that patients should be treated equally and that health care should be accessible to all. Justice should be applied to the way healthcare services are distributed, which means that healthcare services are available to all individuals. Unfortunately, in the United States, the healthcare system does not provide accessibility to all of its citizens. Access to health care is often determined by the ability to pay either out of pocket or by an employer- or government-sponsored program. In countries with universal healthcare coverage, justice in the healthcare industry is more prevalent.

Ethics in the workplace must be governed by the organizational ethics. Ethics has several individual interpretations, so establishing a code of ethics, developing ethics roundtables, creating a decision model for healthcare dilemmas, and providing ongoing ethical training are tools that both HR and management can use to create an ethical culture.

■ Decision Model for Healthcare Dilemmas

Healthcare dilemmas require guidelines to process a solution to the dilemma. Codes of ethics and HR training can assist with a solution. HR training can include a decision-making model that will assist the individual to process the steps in resolving the situation. The following is an adapted version of the steps of the PLUS ethical decision-making model:

1. Identification of the dilemma.
2. Identification of the conflicting ethics of each party.
3. Identification of alternatives to a solution.
4. Identification of the impact of each alternative.
5. Selection of the solution.
6. Evaluation of the solution (PLUS Decision Making Model, 2011).

Application of PLUS Decision-Making Model

Healthcare Dilemma (discussed earlier): An oncologist has a patient who has an advanced stage of melanoma (skin cancer). Prognosis: 3–6 months to live. The oncologist has developed an experimental treatment program that has severe side effects but may give the patient an additional 6 months. The patient prefers alternative remedies for medical treatment such as homeopathic solutions (natural remedies).

Step 1: *Define the problem.* This is the most important part of the process. This step should define the problem and the ultimate outcome of the decision-making process.

Application: The problem is the differing views of treatment by both the physician and the patient. The physician does not believe in homeopathic remedies. The ultimate outcome of the decision-making process is to prolong the life of the patient if possible.

Step 2: *Identify the alternative(s) to the problem*. List the possible alternatives to the desired outcome. Attempt to identify at least three as a minimum, but five are preferred.

Alternative 1: Patient accepts experimental treatment program.

Alternative 2: Patient rejects experimental treatment program.

Alternative 3: Physician researches homeopathic remedies for patient.

Alternative 4: Physician refuses to research homeopathic remedies for patient.

Alternative 5: Patient seeks other medical advice from different physician.

Alternative 6: Physician refers patient to physician who is expert in homeopathic medicine.

Step 3: *Evaluate the identified alternatives*. Discuss the positive and negative impact of each alternative.

Alternative 1: Patient accepts experimental treatment program.

Positive: Patient's cancer is eradicated or is in remission.

Negative: Treatment has no impact on cancer. Patient dies.

Alternative 2: Patient rejects experimental treatment program.

Positive: Cancer goes into remission.

Negative: Patient dies shortly.

Alternative 3: Physician researches homeopathic remedies for patient.

Positive: Physician finds a homeopathic remedy that can be used in conjunction with experimental program. Patient accepts treatment. Cancer is eradicated or goes into remission.

Negative: Physician finds no homeopathic solution that can be used in conjunction with experimental program. Patient refuses treatment. Patient dies shortly.

Alternative 4: Physician refuses to research homeopathic remedies for patient.

Positive: Patient believes in physician and agrees to try experimental program. Program is successful.

Negative: Patient cuts ties with physician. Receives no treatment and dies shortly.

Alternative 5: Patient seeks other medical advice from different physician.

Positive: Patient finds a physician that agrees with homeopathic remedies. Accepts homeopathic remedies and cancer is eradicated or goes into remission.

Negative: Patient does not find a physician who would help her and dies quickly while trying to find someone.

Alternative 6: Physician refers patient to a physician who is an expert in homeopathic medicine.

Positive: Patient is treated with a homeopathic solution that prolongs her life.

Negative: Patient is treated with a homeopathic solution that does not prolong her life.

Step 4: *Make the decision.* In the healthcare industry, the decision must include the patient's best interest and his or her values, which can be conflicting at times. However, the patient has the right to make an informed decision about his or her health.

In this instance, alternative 6 is chosen, because the patient believes in homeopathic medicine. The physician who does not believe in natural remedies respected the patient's beliefs, which differed from hers, but she still wanted to help the patient. The physician wanted to be involved in the patient care by supporting the beliefs of her patient.

Step 5: *Implement the decision.* Once the decision is made, the physician actually finds a physician referral that would help her patient. The primary physician said she would provide any assistance with pain medication if needed.

Step 6: *Evaluate the decision.* An evaluation component of any decision will provide data to assess if the decision was successful in resolving the ethical situation. An evaluation process for this model would be to assess the success of the chosen treatment. Success parameters would be the longevity of the patient's life or the quality of the life of the patient.

This was an actual case. The patient accepted the referral of the new physician and entered a homeopathic treatment program. The patient lived 3 more years with a high quality of life. This decision-making model is an excellent method of resolving many types of healthcare dilemmas. This model can be used in HR training on ethical issues in the healthcare workplace.

■ Codes of Ethics and the Doctor–Patient Relationship

The foundation of health care is the relationship between the patient and physician. As a result of many public ethical crises that have occurred, particularly in the business world, many organizations have developed codes of ethics. **Codes of ethics** provide a standard for operation so that all participants understand that if they do not adhere to this code, there may be negative consequences. The healthcare industry is no different. Physicians have been guided by many healthcare codes of ethics. The American Medical

Association, the professional membership organization for physicians, created a Code of Medical Ethics for physicians in 1847, which has been updated over the years. In 2001, the Code of Medical Ethics was amended to include the following: provide competent medical care, uphold professional standards, respect the law, respect the rights of patients and colleagues, maintain a commitment to medical education, support public health activities, regard patient care as the primary goal, and support medical care access for all individuals (Medical Ethics, 2011). In 2000 and 2001, the **American College of Physicians and Harvard Pilgrim Health Care Ethics Program** developed a statement of ethics for managed care. The following is a summary of the statements:

- Clinicians, healthcare plans, insurance companies, and patients should be honest in their relationship with each other.
- These parties should recognize the importance of the clinician and patient relationship and, in addition, its ethical obligations.
- Clinicians should maintain accurate patient records.
- All parties should contribute to developing healthcare policies.
- The clinician's primary duty is the care of the patient.
- A clinician has the responsibility to practice effective and efficient medicine.
- Clinicians should recognize that all individuals, regardless of their position, should have health care.
- Healthcare plans and their insurers should openly explain their policies regarding reimbursement of types of health care.
- Patients have a responsibility to understand their health insurance.
- Healthcare plans should not ask clinicians to compromise their ethical standards of care.
- Clinicians should enter agreements with healthcare plans that support ethical standards.
- Confidentiality of patient information should be protected.
- Clinicians should disclose conflicts of interest to their patients.
- Information provided to patients should be clearly understood by the patient (Povar et al., 2004).

This statement was developed as a result of the continued economic and policy changes in the healthcare industry. It provided guidelines to healthcare practitioners, to healthcare organizations, and to the healthcare insurance industry about ethical actions in the changing healthcare environment.

■ Other Healthcare Codes of Ethics

Each type of healthcare professional generally has a code of conduct. The American Nurses Association established a code for nurses in 1985, which was revised in 1995 and most recently in 2001 (American Nurses Association, 2011). Healthcare executives have a code of ethics that was established in 1941 that describes the relationship with their stakeholders and that was most recently updated in 2007. The American College of Healthcare Executives represents 30,000 executives internationally who participate in the healthcare system. They established a code of ethics in 1941, which was most recently updated in 2007. They also offer ethical policy statements on relevant issues such as creating an ethical culture for employees. They also offer an ethics self-assessment tool that enables employees to target potential areas of ethical weakness. Many hospitals have also established codes of ethics to help providers when they are dealing with healthcare dilemmas (American College of Healthcare Executives, 2010).

■ How to Develop a Code of Ethics

A code of ethics must be written clearly because employees at all organizational levels will use it. If a certain employee category needs a specific code of ethics, then a written code should be specifically developed for that category. The code must be current in laws and regulations. Driscoll and Hoffman (2000) recommend the following outline for developing a code of ethics:

1. Memorable title
2. Leadership letter
3. Table of contents
4. Introduction
5. Core values of the organization
6. Code provisions
7. Information and resources

The code of ethics must be a user-friendly resource for the organization. It should be updated to include current laws and regulations. The language should be specific as to what the organization should expect from its employees. The organization should provide training on the code of ethics so employees understand the organization's expectations.

■ Ethics and Research

The conduct of research involving human subjects requires assessment of the risks and benefits to the human subjects, which must be explained clearly to them before the consent to participate in the research is given. The principles of ethical research are monitored by **institutional review boards** (IRBs). An IRB is a group that has been formally designated to review and monitor medical research involving human subjects. An IRB has the authority to approve, require modifications in (to secure approval), or disapprove research. This group review serves an important role in the protection of the rights and welfare of human research subjects (Food and Drug Administration, 2009). Any organization that performs research should develop an IRB for their organization. The ethical component of an IRB is to protect the participants of the study. IRBs require researchers to minimize the risks and maximize the benefits to the participant and to explain these assessments clearly. It is important that an IRB not approve a study that imposes significant risks on the subjects.

Assuming the study clears the IRB's assessment of risks and benefits, it is important that the subject understands the study and its impact on him or her. **Research informed consent** is one of the basic ethical protections for human subject research. Informed consent protects human subjects because it allows the individual to consider personal issues before participating in medical research. Informed consent increases autonomy because it provides the individual with the opportunity to make a choice to exercise control over his or her life by disclosing the appropriate information to inform the individual involved in project participation (Mehlman & Berg, 2008). Both the U.S. Department of Health and Human Services and the Food and Drug Administration have outlined common rule regulations that comprise the elements of informed consent.

Common rule elements include a written statement that includes the purpose and duration of the study, the procedures and if they are experimental, any foreseen risks and potential benefits, and any alternative procedures that may benefit the subject (Food and Drug Administration, 2009; Korenman, 2009). Additional requirements are needed for children, pregnant women, people with disabilities, mentally disabled people, prisoners, and so forth. It is clear that the IRB must provide guidelines for parents that have children participating in research and for those subjects that may be mentally disabled who could be unduly influenced (Mehlman & Berg, 2008). It is important that all researchers be trained in IRB protocols to protect themselves, the participants, and the organization.

■ Workplace Bullying—An International Issue

In 1992, Andrea Adams, a BBC journalist, coined the term **"workplace bullying"** to describe an ongoing harassing workplace behavior between employees, which can result in negative outcomes for the targeted employees (Adams, 1992). Workplace bullying is receiving increased attention worldwide as a negative organizational issue. It is considered a serious and chronic workplace stressor that can lead to diminished work productivity and work quality (Namie & Namie, 2009). Although the definitions are similar worldwide, there are different labels of bullying that are used—mobbing is used in France and Germany, harassment in Finland, and in the United States and Australia, aggression, emotional abuse, or workplace bullying (Sheehan, 1999; Keashly, 2001). Research in Scandinavian countries indicates that bullying prevalence rates range from 3.5% to 16%, with United Kingdom research reporting higher prevalence rates (Privitera, Psych & Campbell, 2009).

This negative behavior is considered bullying if it is repeated over an extended period of time. It can occur between colleagues, supervisors, or supervisees, although the bully is often the supervisor. Definitions also include negative verbal or nonverbal behavior such as snide comments, verbal or physical threats, or items being thrown. Employees have also reported less aggressive behavior such as someone demeaning their work or gossiping about them on a continual basis. The literature has reported an increased incidence of bullying reported in healthcare organizations and in academe (Vartia, 2001; Ayoko, Callan & Hartel, 2003; Djurkovic, McCormack & Casimir, 2008).

Workplace Bullying in Health Care

Workplace bullying is common in health care. Specifically, there are bullying issues between physicians and nurses. A 2004 survey by the Institute for Safe Medication Practices indicated that of the 2,095 respondents, which included nurses, pharmacists, and other providers, more than 50% were verbally abused by physicians when asking for clarification regarding prescription orders. The Center for American Nurses, American Association of Critical-Care Nurses, International Council of Nurses, and National Student Nurses Association have all issued statements regarding the need for healthcare organizations to stop bullying in the healthcare workplace. Often, verbal abuse also occurs toward nurses by physicians, patients, and families of patients. **Lateral violence** also occurs in health care, which is defined as "nurse to nurse" aggression, demonstrated by both verbal and nonverbal behavior (Lateral Violence and Bullying in the Workplace, 2011).

Workplace Bullying Institute

The Workplace Bullying Institute was started in the 1990s in the United States by Dr. Gary and Ruth Nanie as a result of Ruth being bullied in her workplace by a female supervisor. They established a website (http://www.workplacebullying .org) in 2002 as a venue to promote and educate the public on workplace bullying. In August 2007, they conducted the first study of all adult Americans on workplace bullying—the results indicating that workplace bullying was a major organizational issue. Approximately 8,000 respondents, representative of the U.S. adult population, indicated that 37% of the workers were bullied. Approximately 70% of the bullying was from supervisors with 60% of those bullies being women. The women bullies targeted women in 71% of the cases. According to the survey, more than 60% of the employers ignored the problem. It was also reported by 45% of those who were bullied that they experienced stress-related health problems such as anxiety, depression, and panic attacks (Workplace Bullying, 2011). These results are consistent with reports from the literature.

Impact of Workplace Bullying

As indicated earlier, workplace bully targets can experience a range of physical and psychological symptoms such as work stress anxiety, lowered job satisfaction and loyalty to the organization, increase in absenteeism, lowered work productivity, and depression (Ayoko et al., 2003). A sense of powerlessness is often reported by the target. In order for a bully to be successful, the target must feel that he or she cannot defend himself or herself against the bully, which allows the bully to continue the behavior. In two Australian studies, more than 40% of the employees were bullied by their supervisors, more than 10% were bullied by their peers, and 2% were bullied by their subordinates (Ayoko et al., 2003).

Workplace bullying also affects other employees because if the bullying continues and is not addressed by management, it affects the overall morale of the workforce. Low morale often results in high employee turnover, which can be detrimental to the organization's success. It also can disrupt the professional career of the target as well as the personal life of the target. From an organizational perspective, continued bullying may result in the organization paying for litigation fees, counseling, workers' compensation, and early retirement payouts (Kieseker & Merchant, 1999).

Legal Implications of Workplace Bullying

Unfortunately, 80% of workplace bullying incidents is not illegal. There is no specific legislation in the United States that forbids workplace bullying. Thirteen states have introduced bills. New York is the only state that has enacted legislation that forbids this type of behavior in the workplace. There are two federal laws that can be applied in workplace bullying: the Occupational Safety and Health Act of 1970 and Title VII of the Civil Rights Act of 1964. Under the Occupational Safety and Health Act of 1970, the employer must provide a safe and healthful working environment for its employees. Under Title VII of the Civil Rights Act, if a protected class employee (gender, religion, ethnicity, etc.) is bullied by another employee, the action can be illegal based on the concept of a hostile work environment, which is illegal under sexual harassment.

Recommendations to Eliminate Workplace Bullying

To date, there is no federal legislation that specifically addresses workplace bullying. To reduce the prevalence of workplace bullying, it is important that employers implement policies to eliminate this behavior. The following are recommendations for organizations including healthcare organizations:

1. Adopt a policy of zero tolerance for workplace bullying and develop measures to discipline bullies in the workplace.

2. Create an organizational culture that focuses on a positive work environment enabling all individuals to pursue their careers.
3. Reward behaviors that encourage teamwork and collaboration among employees and their supervisors.
4. Develop an educational program for all employees on what constitutes workplace bullying (LaVan & Martin, 2007).

Workplace bullying continues to be a pervasive organizational problem worldwide. In the United States, the Workplace Bullying Institute has developed a Healthy Workplace Bill that precisely defines workplace bullying and extends protection to employees against this type of behavior. The bill has been introduced in 14 states since 2003. There is no specific federal legislation against bullying, so bullying will unfortunately continue to be legal. It is important that workplace bullying educational programs and organizational policies be implemented to ensure that employees will be protected against this type of negative behavior. The results can be devastating from both an organizational and individual level.

In 2008, the Joint Commission developed a standard for workplace bullying that they call intimidating and disruptive behaviors in the workplace. They issued the following statement:

> Intimidating and disruptive behaviors can foster medical errors, contribute to poor patient satisfaction and to preventable adverse outcomes, increase the cost of care, and cause qualified clinicians, administrators, and managers to seek new positions in more professional environments. Safety and quality of patient care is dependent on teamwork, communication, and a collaborative work environment. To assure quality and to promote a culture of safety, health care organizations must address the problem of behaviors that threaten the performance of the health care team.

Two leadership standards are now part of the Joint Commission's accreditation provisions: The first requires an institution to have "a code of conduct that defines acceptable and disruptive and inappropriate behaviors." The second requires an institution "to create and implement a process for managing disruptive and inappropriate behaviors" (Yamada, 2011).

In a recent Joint Commission study, it was found that more than 50% of nurses have suffered some type of bullying, with 90% observing some type of abuse. Their standard focused on the impact of these types of behavior on patient care quality. The Joint Commission requires healthcare institutions to create a code of conduct that defines appropriate behavior and has a system in place to manage inappropriate behavior such as workplace bullying. In addition to the stance of the Joint Commission, the Center for Professional Health at the Vanderbilt University Medical Center has developed a program for treating and remediating disruptive behaviors by physicians. Nurses' unions are also developing education programs on workplace bullying (Minding the Workplace, 2011).

Conclusion

The HR department must provide training for all employees to ensure that they understand the seriousness of violating the law and understand the differences between civil and criminal law and the penalties that may be imposed for breaking those laws. Both federal and state laws have been enacted and policy has been implemented to protect both the healthcare provider and the healthcare consumer. New laws have been passed and older laws have been amended to reflect needed changes regarding health care to continue to protect its participants.

In the healthcare industry, there are several areas of operation that are affected by ethics. Healthcare ethical dilemmas develop between providers and patients when there may be a conflict of personal ethical standards. If research is performed by an organization and its employees, IRB training must be implemented to ensure that ethical guidelines are followed when performing research on humans.

Workplace bullying has become an international workplace issue. At this time, there is no federal mandate that targets this type of behavior. Statistics indicate that this behavior is occurring in the healthcare workplace. HR training must target this type of unethical behavior. Developing and enforcing a code of ethics provides a standard for operation so that all participants understand that if they do not adhere to this code, there may be negative consequences.

Vocabulary

Affirmative action plan
Age Discrimination in Employment
    Act of 1967
American College of Physicians and
    Harvard Pilgrim Health Care
    Ethics Program
Americans with Disabilities Act
Assault
Autonomy
Battery
Beneficence
Carpal tunnel syndrome
Civil law
Civil Rights Act of 1964
Civil Rights Act of 1991
Codes of ethics
Common law

Common rule
Compensatory damages
Consolidated Omnibus Budget
    Reconciliation Act
Criminal law
Defensive medicine
Employee Retirement Income
    Security Act
Equal Pay Act
Ergonomics
Essential functions
Ethical standards
Ethics
Family Medical Leave Act
General duty
Genetic Information
    Nondiscrimination Act

Hazard Communication standard
Health care ethical dilemma
Health Insurance Portability and
  Accountability Act
HIPAA National Standards
Informed consent
Intellectual disabilities
Intentional torts
Institutional review boards
Invasion of privacy
Job lock
Justice
Lateral violence
Law
Lilly Ledbetter Fair Pay Act
Material Safety Data Sheets
Medical malpractice
Mental Health Parity Act
Monetary cap
National Defense Authorization Act
Negligence
No malfeasance
Occupational Safety and Health Act

Older Workers Benefit Protection
  Act
Patient Protection and Affordable
  Care Act
Pension Protection Act
Personal protective equipment
Pregnancy Discrimination Act
Punitive damage
Rehabilitation Act
Research informed consent
Rules and regulations
Sexual harassment
Standard of care
Statutes
Tort reform
Torts
Uniformed Services Employment
  and Reemployment Rights Act
Voluntary hospital
Wellstone Act
Worker Adjustment and Retraining
  Notification Act
Workplace bullying

■ References

Adams, A. (1992). *Bullying at Work*. London, UK: Vrago Press, pp. 1–20.

American College of Healthcare Executives Code of Ethics (2011). Available at: http://www.advamed .org/MemberPortal/About/code/. Accessed February 2, 2011.

American Heritage Dictionary (2000). Boston, MA: Houghton Mifflin, p. 1060.

American Medical Association (2010). Code of Ethics. Available at: http://www.ama-assn.org/ ama/pub/physician-resources/medical-ethics/code-medical-ethics/. Accessed November 10, 2010.

American Nurses Association (2011). Nursing World. Available at: http://www.nursingworld.org/ MainMenuCategories/EthicsStandards.aspx. Accessed January 5, 2011.

Americans with Disabilities Act of 1990 (2011). Available at: http://www.ada.gov/pubs/ada.htm. Accessed December 3, 2011.

Anderson, R., Rice, T., & Kominski, G. (2007). Changing the U.S. Healthcare system. San Francisco, CA: Jossey-Boss.

Ayoko, O., Callan, V. & Hartel, C. (2003). Workplace conflict, bullying and counterproductive behaviors. *International Journal of Organizational Analysis*, 11:283–301.

Beauchamp, T. & Childress, J. (2001). *Principles of Biomedical Ethics* (5th ed.). Oxford, UK: Oxford University Press.

Buchbinder, S. & Shanks, N. (2007). *Introduction to Health Care Management*. Sudbury, MA: Jones & Bartlett Learning, p. 347–48.

Danzon, P. (1995). *Medical Malpractice: Theory, Evidence, and Public Policy*. Cambridge, MA: Harvard University Press.

Department of Labor. (2011). Available at: http://www.dol.gov/ebsa/Regs/fedreg/final/2006009557 .htm. Accessed June 1, 2011.

Djurkovic, N., McCormack, D. & Casimir, G. (2008). Workplace bullying and intention to leave: The modernizing effect of perceived organizational support. *Human Resource Management Journal*, 18(4):405–420.

Drachsler, D. (2010). Notes on: Year one of the Lilly Ledbetter Fair Pay Act. *Labor Law Journal*, Summer 2010:102–106.

Driscoll, D. & Hoffman, W. (2000). *Ethics Matters: How to Implement Values-Driven Management*. Waltham, MA: Center for Business Ethics at Bentley College, pp. 70–80.

Einarsen, S., Hoel, H., Zapf, D. & Cooper, C. L. (2003). The concept of bullying at work: the European tradition. In: *Bullying and Emotional Abuse in the Workplace: International Perspectives in Research and Practice*. 1st ed. London: Taylor & Francis, p 3-30.

Emanuel, E. (2008). *Health Care Guaranteed*. New York, NY: Public Affairs.

Food and Drug Administration (2009). Information Sheet Guidance for Institutional Review Boards, Clinical Investigators, and Sponsors. Available at: http://www.fda.gov/oc/ohrt/irbs/facts .html#IRBOrg. Accessed November 4, 2010.

Gillon, R. (1994) Principles of medical ethics. *British Medical Journal*, 309:184.

Gomez-Mejia, L., Balkin, D. & Cardy, R. (2012). *Managing Human Resources*. Upper Saddle River, NJ: Pearson, pp. 100–125.

Hickman, J., Gilligan, M. & Patton, G. (2008). FMLA and benefit obligations: New rights under an old mandate. *Benefits Law Journal*, 21(3):5–16.

Keashly, L. (2001). Interpersonal and systemic aspects of emotional abuse at work: The target's perspective. *Violence and Victims,* 16:233–268.

Kieseker, R. & Merchant, T. (1999). Workplace bullying in Australia: A review of current conceptualizations and research. *Australian Journal of Management and Organizational Behavior*, 2: 61–75.

Kolpack, D., (2010). PPACA's adult child coverage requirement clarified. Available at: https://www .bcbsnd.com/blueinsight/2010/04/12/ppaca%E2%80%99s-adult-child-coverage-requirement-clarified/. Accessed December 3, 2011.

Korenman, S. G. (2010). Teaching the responsible conduct of research in humans. Available at: http:// ori.hhs.gov/education/products/ucla/chapter2/page04b.htm. Accessed November 4, 2010.

Lateral Violence and Bullying in the Workplace (2011). Available at: http://www.tnaonline.org/Media/ pdf/wkpl-viol-dec-10-can-conflict-bully-fact-sheet.pdf. Accessed December 3, 2011.

LaVan, H. & Martin, W. (2007). Bullying in the U.S. workplace: Normative and process-oriented ethical approaches. *Journal of Business Ethics*, 83:147–165.

Medical Ethics (2011). Available at: http://www.ama-assn.org/ama/pub/physician-resources/medical-ethics/code-medical-ethics.page?. Accessed July 7, 2011.

Medical Negligence: The role of America's civil justice system in protecting patient rights (2011). American Association for Justice. Available at: http://www.kff.org/insurance/upload/Medical-Malpractice-Law-in-the-United-States-Report.pdf. Accessed December 3, 2011.

Mehlman, M. & Berg, J. (2008). Human subjects' protections in biomedical enhancement research: Assessing risk and benefit and obtaining informed consent. *Journal of Law, Medicine & Ethics,* Fall:546–559.

Miller, R. (2006a). *Problems in Health Care Law* (9th ed.). Sudbury, MA: Jones and Bartlett Publishers, p. 1.

Miller, R. (2006b). *Problems in Health Care Law* (9th ed.). Sudbury, MA: Jones and Bartlett Publishers, p. 686.

Miller, R. (2006c). *Problems in Health Care Law* (9th ed.). Sudbury, MA: Jones and Bartlett Publishers, p. 605.

Miller, R. (2006d). *Problems in Health Care Law* (9th ed.). Sudbury, MA: Jones and Bartlett Publishers, p. 586.

Miller, R. (2006e). *Problems in Health Care Law* (9th ed.). Sudbury, MA: Jones and Bartlett Publishers, p. 587.

Miller, R. (2006f). *Problems in Health Care Law* (9th ed.). Sudbury, MA: Jones and Bartlett Publishers, p. 341.

Minding the Workplace (2011). Available at: http://neworkplace.wordpress.com/2009/12/15/workplace-bullying-in-healthcare. Accessed June 10, 2011.

Namie, G. & Namie, R (2009). U.S. workplace bullying: Some basic considerations and consultation interventions. *Consulting Psychology Journal,* 61 (3), 202–219.National Human Genome Research Institute (2011). Available at: http://www.genome.gov/About/. Accessed March 1, 2011.

Nelson III, L., Morrisey, M. & Kilgore, M. (2007). Damages caps in malpractice cases. *The Milbank Quarterly,* 85(2):259–286.

Niles, N. (2010). *Basics of the U.S. Health Care System.* Sudbury, MA: Jones & Bartlett, pp. 247–259.

Noe, R., Hollenbeck, J., Gerhart, B. & Wright, P. (2009). *Fundamentals of Human Resource Management* (3rd ed.). Boston, MA: McGraw-Hill/Irwin.

Occupational Safety & Health Administration (2010). *Ergonomics.* Retrieved from http://www.osha.gov/SLTC/ergonomics/. Accessed April 1, 2011.

Office of Technology Assessment (1993). *Impact of Legal Reforms on Medical Malpractice Cost,* OTA-BP-H-19. Washington, DC: U.S. Government Printing Office.

PLUS Decision Making Model (2011). Available at: http://www.ethics.org/resource/plus-decision-making-model. Accessed September 22, 2011.

Povar, C., Blumen, H., Daniel, J., Daub, S., Evans, L., Holm, R., et al. (2004). Ethics in practice: Obama, Task Force call on Senate to pass Paycheck Fairness Act. *Bureau of National Affairs,* September 2010:11–14.

Privitera, C., Psych, M. & Campbell, M. (2009). Cyberbullying: The new face of workplace bullying? *Cyber Psychology & Behavior,* 12(4):395–400.

Rosenbach, M. & Stone, A. (1990). Malpractice insurance costs and physician practice—1981–1986. *Health Affairs,* 9:176–185.

Sedhom, S. (2009). Reacting to the Lilly Ledbetter Fair Pay Act: What every employer needs to know. *Employee Relations Law Journal,* 35(3):3–8.

Sheehan, M. (1999). Workplace bullying: Responding with some emotional intelligence. *International Journal of Manpower,* 20(1/2):57–69.

Shi, L. & Singh, D. (2008a). *Essentials of the U.S. Health Care Delivery System.* Sudbury, MA: Jones and Bartlett Publishers, p. 17.

Shi, L. & Singh, D. (2008b). *Essentials of the U.S. Health Care Delivery System*. Sudbury, MA: Jones and Bartlett Publishers, p. 227.

Stanwyck, P. & Stanwyck, S. (2009). *Understanding Business Ethics*. Upper Saddle River, NJ: Pearson Prentic Hall, pp. 110–112.

Sultz, H. & Young, K. (2006). Healthcare USA: Understanding its organization and delivery. Sudbury, MA: Jones and Bartlett Publishers.

Taylor, P. (1975). *Principles of Ethics: An Introduction to Ethics* (2nd ed.). Encino, CA: Dickinson.

The Privacy Rule (2011). Available at: http://www.hhs.gov/ocr/privacy/hipaa/administrative/privacyrule/index.html. Accessed December 3, 2011.

Vartia, M. (2001). Consequences of workplace bullying with respect to the well-being of its targets and the observers of bullying. *Scandinavian Journal of Work Environment and Health*, 27:63–59.

Waters, T., Budetti, P., Claxton, G. & Lundy, J. (2007). Impact of state tort reforms on physician malpractice payments. *Health Affairs*, 26(2):500–509.

Workplace Bullying (2011). Available at: http://www.workplacebulllying.org. Accessed July 7, 2011.

Wynia, M. (2007). Ethics and public health emergencies: Encouraging responsibility. *The American Journal of Bioethics*, 7:1–4.

Yamada, D. (2011). *Workplace Bullying in Healthcare: The Joint Commission Standards*. Available at: http://newworkplace.wordpress.com/2009/12/15/workplace-bullying-in-healthcare-i-the-joint-commission-standards/. Accessed September 23, 2011.

STUDENT WORKBOOK ACTIVITY 2.1

Complete the following case scenarios based on the information provided in this chapter. Your answer must be *in your own words*.

Real-Life Applications: Case Scenario 1

As the HR new employee trainer, you are in charge of orientation for four new employees regarding employment law. There is one female, one disabled, one African American, and one Muslim individual. You believe it is important to emphasize laws that were passed to protect employees from discrimination.

Activity

Select the laws you believe are the most important to the new employees. Provide a brief description of each law and its impact on the new employees.

Responses

_____

_____

_____

_____

_____

_____

_____

_____

_____

_____

_____

_____

_____

_____

_____

_____

_____

_____

_____

_____

Real-Life Applications: Case Scenario 2

The CEO of your managed care organization has asked you to discuss the importance of ethics in the workplace. He has requested that you develop mandatory ethics training for all employees. Your CEO specifically asked that you address any ethics codes that target managed care.

Activity

Devise an ethics training that includes healthcare codes of ethics for managed care. Also, suggest five ways to improve ethics in the managed care organization.

Responses

_____

_____

_____

_____

_____

_____

_____

_____

_____

_____

_____

_____

_____

_____

_____

_____

_____

Real-Life Applications: Case Scenario 3

As the new manager of the local public health department, you want to be sure that your employees understand their roles in the department and how they should interact with individuals when providing public health interventions.

Activity

Design a program that focuses on ethics in the public health workplace.

Responses

_____

_____

_____

_____

_____

_____

_____

_____

_____

_____

_____

_____

_____

_____

_____

Real-Life Applications: Case Scenario 4

You have been experiencing some negative behavior from a physician you are working with and your nursing supervisor. You are not sure what to do. You decide to go to HR to find out what can be done to rectify these problems.

Activity

You speak to the HR department to find out more about bullying and lateral violence and what the organization can do to rectify these ongoing problems. Please provide the information you found from HR.

Responses

_____

_____

_____

_____

_____

_____

_____

_____

_____

_____

_____

_____

_____

_____

_____

_____

_____

_____

_____

STUDENT WORKBOOK ACTIVITY 2.2

In Your Own Words

Based on this chapter, please provide an explanation of the following concepts in your own words as they apply to human resource management. *Do not recite* the text.

Criminal law:

_____

_____

_____

Civil law:

_____

_____

_____

Healthcare ethical dilemma:

_____

_____

_____

Autonomy:

_____

_____

_____

Workplace bullying:

_____

_____

_____

Torts:

_____

_____

_____

Lateral violence:

_____

_____

_____

Job lock:

_____

_____

_____

Defensive medicine:

_____

_____

_____

STUDENT WORKBOOK ACTIVITY 2.3

Internet Exercises

Write your answers in the spaces provided.

- Visit each of the websites listed in the text that follows.
- Name the organization.
- Locate its mission statement on its website.
- Provide a brief overview of the activities of the organization.
- Apply this organization to the chapter information.

Websites
http://www.justice.gov

Organization name:

_____

Mission statement:

_____

_____

_____

Overview of activities:

_____

_____

_____

Application to chapter information:

_____

_____

_____

http://www.genome.gov

Organization name:

_____

Mission statement:

_____

_____

_____

Overview of activities:

_____

_____

_____

Application to chapter information:

_____

_____

_____

http://www.healthlaw.org

Organization name:

_____

Mission statement:

_____

_____

_____

Overview of activities:

_____

_____

_____

Application to chapter information:

_____

_____

_____

http://www.eeoc.gov

Organization name:

_____

Mission statement:

_____

_____

_____

Overview of activities:

_____

_____

_____

Application to chapter information:

_____

_____

_____

http://www.workplacebullying.org

Organization name:

_____

Mission statement:

_____

_____

_____

Overview of activities:

_____

_____

_____

Application to chapter information:

_____

_____

_____

http://www.abanet.org

Organization name:

_____

Mission statement:

_____

_____

_____

Overview of activities:

_____

_____

_____

Application to chapter information:

_____

_____

_____

STUDENT ACTIVITY 2.4: DISCUSSION BOARDS FOR ONLINE, HYBRID, AND TRADITIONAL ONGROUND CLASSES

Discussion Board Guidelines

The discussion board is used in online and web-enhanced courses in place of classroom lectures and discussion. The board can be an enhancement to traditional onground classes. The discussion board is the way in which the students "link together" as a class. The following are guidelines to help focus on the discussion topic and to define the roles and responsibilities of the discussion coordinator and other members of the class. The educator will be the discussion moderator for this course.

1. The educator will post the discussion topic and directions for the upcoming week. These postings should all be responses to the original topic or responses to other students' responses. When people respond to what someone else has posted, they should start the posting with the person's name so it is clear which

message they are responding to. **A response such as "Yes" or "I agree" does not count for credit. Your responses must be in your own words. You cannot copy and paste from the text.**

2. Postings (especially responses) should include enough information so the message is clear but should not be so long that it becomes difficult to follow. Remember, this is like talking to someone in a classroom setting. The postings should reflect the content of the text or other assignments. If you retrieve information from the Internet, the hyperlink must be cited.

3. Students should check the discussion daily to see if new information has been posted that requires their attention and response.

Good discussion will often include different points of view. Students should feel free to disagree or "challenge" others to support their positions or ideas. All discussions must be handled in a respectful manner. The following are discussion boards for this chapter.

Discussion Boards

1. Discuss the concepts of negligence and intentional torts, and give examples of these in the healthcare industry.
2. What is tort reform? Do you believe tort reform is necessary?
3. Discuss three employment-related pieces of legislation that you believe are very important and why.
4. What is your definition of ethics? What do you think are some unethical situations in the healthcare industry?

Staffing the Organization

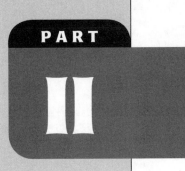

PART

II

Designing Jobs

DID YOU KNOW THAT?

- Job analysis is the foundation of human resource management because the analysis of a job is required before an organization recruits individuals for specific positions.
- Micromotion such as holding an object is the simplest unit of work.
- Two or more micromotions become an element such as holding or taking an object.
- An excellent external resource for obtaining statistics about healthcare labor is the U.S. Department of Labor.
- The Americans with Disabilities Act of 1990 requires organizations to identify the essential job functions or ensure that disabled individuals can be included in a job recruitment process to ensure that such individuals can perform the major job activities in a position, reducing the possibility of discrimination.

■ Introduction

When creating an organization, the first task is to determine its overall goal or mission. If the goal is long-term care, for example, then the first major decision is to decide how the activities flow through the organization. If a healthcare organization changes its services, workflow analysis must be repeated. For example, more healthcare organizations are using more technology in their operations such as electronic patient health records. Implementation of this type of transition would necessitate a workflow review to ensure that this new requirement would be successful.

Evaluating the workflow of any organization is the first step to developing jobs for individuals. This first step ensures the workflow produces the desired outputs of an organization. Once the workflow is analyzed, the next step is to design jobs for employees who will be responsible for producing the output of the organization. This chapter will discuss workflow, workflow analysis, job analysis, job designs and job redesigns, job descriptions and specifications, and the resources available to accomplish these necessary tasks.

■ Workflow Analysis of an Organization (Inputs, Activity, Outputs)

Workflow is the activities that combine the processes, tools, and labor working toward achieving the stated goal of an organization. Workflow generally consists of several steps of activity from different labor points (Essex, 2000). **Workflow analysis** analyzes these activities through an organization. The first step of workflow analysis is to identify the outputs or goal of an organization. Healthcare organizations typically provide services. For example, an output or goal of the organization is to provide long-term care services. The next step in the process is to determine what **work activity** (tasks and jobs) is needed to achieve the **outputs** or services. To achieve the work activity, what **inputs** such as the type of employees, equipment, and information are needed to perform the work activity to achieve the outputs/services? The same process is performed if the organization decides to alter the way a service is offered. For example, if electronic medical records will be implemented in this long-term care organization, the current workflow patterns are redesigned to accommodate the new technology (How Do I perform, 2011).

■ Job Analysis

A **job** is a set of related duties or tasks. The simplest unit of work is a **micromotion** such as holding an object. Two or more micromotions become an **element** such as taking an object. A group of elements becomes a **task** (Byars & Rue, 2006, p. 64). These tasks are the related duties of the job. **Job analysis** is the process of determining which type of related duties is appropriate for a specific job. By determining the types of job duties, a job analysis also assesses the knowledge, skills, and abilities needed to perform the job (Mathis & Jackson, 2006a, p. 171). Job analysis can be performed by observing an individual in the job, interviewing employees, having employees write work diaries about their job duties, or having employees or supervisors complete a questionnaire. Job analysis is the foundation of human resource management because the analysis of a job is required before an organization recruits individuals for specific jobs. At the conclusion of a job analysis, a written job description and written job specifications are developed that outline the responsibilities, skills, and experience needed to perform the job successfully.

How to Perform a Job Analysis

The most important step in performing a job analysis is to collect information about the different types of jobs in a healthcare organization. The information is collected from different sources to ensure that the job analysis is inclusive. A common method is to observe employees in their current jobs to determine the different tasks they perform. A second method is to survey the employees to find out their opinions about their jobs. A structured questionnaire is given to employees to ensure there is reliability when generating consistent employee information. Supervisors are also interviewed to ensure there is objectivity when analyzing jobs. Management can develop its own questionnaires or use existing labor questionnaires such as the **Position Analysis Questionnaire** (PAQ). The PAQ, developed in 1972, is an objective and structured job analysis tool consisting of 195 job elements that generally represent work activities. The PAQ is one of the best quantitative instruments that may be used to analyze jobs. It retrieves information in the following areas: how workers obtain information to perform a job; cognitive activities to perform a job; tools needed to perform a job; the percentage of time spent on individual tasks; what other employees are needed to perform a job; and where the job is located in the organization. The PAQ focuses more on worker performance than on technical aspects of a job. It is used frequently to assess the validity of employee selection processes. Service sector PAQs such as those for the healthcare industry will focus on identifying the most critical tasks performed, the type of support for the employee to complete the tasks, the type of work performed prior to the employee completing his or her tasks, ramifications if work is not completed, and why the employee's job actually exists (ASU PAQ, 2008). Typically, supervisors or job analysts complete the PAQ because the comprehension is at a college level. In addition to PAQs, a **Management Position Description Questionnaire** is also used to assess managerial qualities such as decision making and supervision (Mathis & Jackson, 2006b, p. 179). Typically, a job analysis is performed by an outside consultant, by management, or by a job analyst.

Job Analyst's Role

A **job analyst** or personnel analyst is located in the human resources (HR) department of an organization. According to the O*NET, a job analyst collects, analyzes, and prepares occupational information about specific jobs and collaborates with management to develop job descriptions and job specifications. The job analyst may analyze jobs by observing and interviewing appropriate personnel. The analyst provides recommendations to improve recruiting, selecting, promoting, training, and performance appraisal. Job analysts are helpful in this process because they are objective agents for analysis of the activities of employees. Small organizations, however, may not have a designated HR department and may hire a job analyst as an external consultant (Human Resources, 2011). Several approaches are used when performing a job analysis to ensure reliability and validity in the process. Employees and their supervisors could inflate the importance of jobs because they are afraid they may lose their jobs. An employee interview or questionnaire may be very helpful. An organization could hire an outside consultant such as a job analyst to complete this important process.

Importance of Job Analysis

Once a job analysis is performed, the organization must identify the job responsibilities and the job requirements or job specifications. From a legal perspective, the Americans with Disabilities Act of 1990 (ADA) requires organizations to identify the **essential job functions** or the fundamental activities of a position to ensure that individuals who are disabled can be included in a job recruitment process and that they can perform the major job activities in a position (Mathis & Jackson, 2006c, pp. 107–108).

Job analysis can also be used to determine whether an employee is exempt or nonexempt as it pertains to eligibility for overtime. A PAQ is helpful in determining the percentage of time employees spend on management or supervisory activities. If an employee spends more than 50% of his or her time on management and/or supervisory activities, then he or she is exempt and not qualified for overtime pay. In addition, if an employee is considered exempt, he or she may not be eligible for representation in a union's bargaining unit (Fried & Fottler, 2008, pp. 383–384).

U.S. Department of Labor

An excellent external resource for obtaining information about healthcare labor is the U.S. Department of Labor. The Department of Labor provides current statistics about employment, union representation, earnings, and workplace trends for these sectors (About DOL, 2011). It also provides general information on 100 industries including the healthcare and social assistance sector (NAICS 62) and its subsectors of hospitals (NAICS 622), ambulatory healthcare services (NAICS 621), nursing and residential care facilities (NACIS 623), and social assistance (NAICS 624). Established in 1998, the North American Industry Classification System (NAICS) compares economic data across the United States, Canada, and Mexico. Each category is classified by this system to ensure a direct comparison across country borders (What Is NAICS, 2010).

O*NET

In the 1930s, the U.S. Department of Labor developed a Dictionary of Occupational Titles (DOT), which described more than 10,000 jobs. This was replaced in 1998 by the **Occupational Information Network (O*NET),** a website-based application that allows users to review tasks, skills, training, and experience needed for different jobs (O*NET, 2011). Based on information from the Bureau of Labor Statistics, O*NET has identified approximately 100 general healthcare categories of jobs, the tasks associated with the jobs, and their projected growth. O*NET also has established a competency model clearinghouse.

Industry Competency Model

Rather than assessing jobs using the task analysis approach, the industry competency job analysis approach provides an alternative method of assessment. **Competencies** are skills, knowledge, or abilities needed to perform a job or activity in an organization. A competency model organizes the competencies needed to perform in a particular industry. The U.S. Department of Labor's Employment and Training Administration has developed a **competency model** for the long-term care, supports, and services industry. The administration's goal is to provide education to employees who work with the elderly and disabled to encourage independence in their clients' lives. The American Health Care Association, Paraprofessionals Healthcare Institute, College of Direct Support, National Center for Assisted Living, American Network of Community Options and Resources, Institute for the Future of Aging Services, University of Minnesota Institute on Community Integration, University of Alaska, Anchorage for Community Development, and the National Alliance for Direct Support Professionals participated in the development of the competency model.

The Building Blocks Model is a competency model that is viewed as a pyramid. It consists of personal effectiveness competencies; academic, workplace, industry-wide, and industry-sector competencies; occupational-specific knowledge areas; technical requirements; occupational-specific requirements; and management competencies. These areas are considered the building blocks for model development (Figure 3.1). The following is a description of each of the nine tiers of competencies.

> Tier 1: **Personal effectiveness competencies:** They are located at the base of the pyramid and influence the other competencies. These competencies include interpersonal skills, initiative, dependability, and willingness to learn. These represent generic types of traits and motivation that can be applied to many different industries.

> Tier 2: **Academic competencies:** These are located one level above the personal effectiveness competencies and represent critical skills learned from an academic setting. Competencies such as mathematics, reading, writing, and communication apply to many industries.

Tier 3: **Workplace competencies:** These competencies are specific to many industries and include planning and organizing, problem solving, computer proficiency, adaptability, and customer focus.

Tier 4: **Industry-wide technical competencies:** These competencies are generally needed within an industry such as supply chain management, operations, health, and safety.

Tier 5: **Industry-sector technical competencies.** These competencies must be identified by the industry that is assessing the competencies such as the food manufacturing industry.

Tier 6: **Occupation-specific knowledge areas:** These areas are identified in O*NET and include food production, chemistry, sales and marketing, and accounting. O*NET has a large list of these areas. They are customized according to the specific area of the occupation.

Tier 7: **Occupation-specific technical requirements:** Building on level 6, there are technical areas that must be identified by the specific occupation.

Tier 8: **Occupation-specific requirements:** This is the top level of the pyramid and includes certification, licensure, and educational degrees required to obtain certain competencies.

Tier 9: **Management competencies:** These are specific to supervisors and include delegating, networking, motivating and inspiring, and strategic planning (Building Blocks Model, 2010).

Based on the Building Blocks Model, industries such as health care will develop a competency model to perform in the industry. For example, Figure 3.2 is a model for competencies in long-term care and Figure 3.3 is a competency model for electronic health records. Under Tier 1 and Tier 2, each of these industries would select different personal effectiveness and academic competencies that would be important to the long-term care industry. For example, under Tier 1 and 2, both industries select the same personal effectiveness and academic competencies; however, under Tier 2, information literacy was important to the electronic health records industry. Under Tier 3, there continued to be a similar focus on **workplace competencies;** however, long-term care chose instruction and business fundamentals as important to learn. Electronic health records focused on checking, examining, and recording information and workplace fundamentals. The remaining tiers focus on specific competencies needed for each industry. Long-term care focused on long-term care and services, daily living focus, crisis prevention, ethics, and competencies related to accreditation. Electronic health records competencies focused on health information and healthcare delivery, ethics, and health informatics.

These models are interactive, and the user can select which competencies are needed for a specific job. The model contains certain competencies and allows the user to add competencies if needed based on application to different industries or organizations.

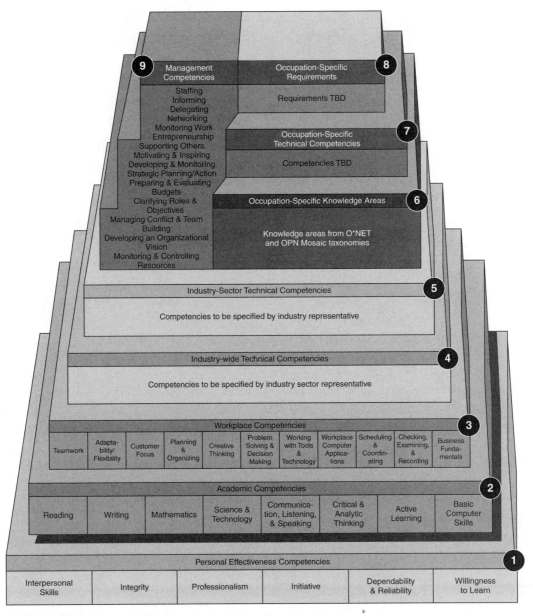

Figure 3.1 Building blocks of the competency model.
Reproduced from: CareerOneStop (2011). Career Competency Models: Geospatial Technology Competency Model. http//:www.careeronestop.org/CompetencyModel/pyramid.aspx. Accessed December 5, 2011.

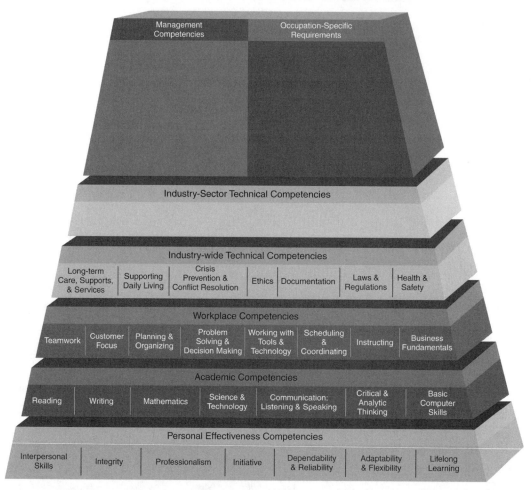

Figure 3.2 Long-term care, supports, and services competency model. Reproduced from: CareerOneStop (2011). Career Competency Models: Long-term Care, Supports, and Services Competency Model. http://www.careeronestop.org/ CompetencyModel/pyramid.aspx?LTC=Y. Accessed December 5, 2011.

Importance of Competencies

These competency models can play an important role in an organization. Organizations develop both short-term goals and long-term goals. Establishment of organizational goals provides a foundation for all employees including management to work together to achieve organizational success. Part of this goal-setting process is to determine the existing competencies of an organization. As stated earlier, competencies are an activity that an organization performs well. Competencies are derived from the employees'

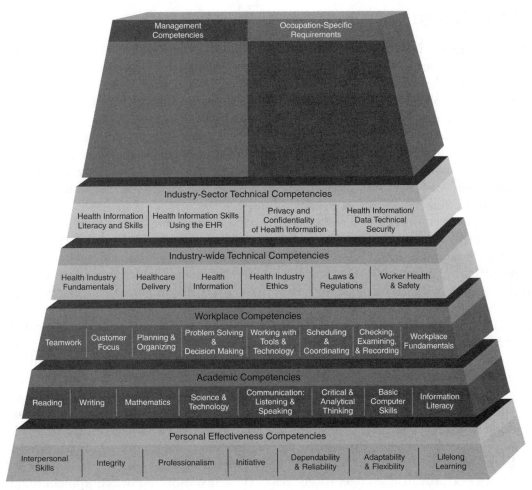

Figure 3.3 Electronic health records competency model.
Reproduced from: CareerOneStop (2011). Career Competency Models: Health: Electronic Health Records Competency Model. http://www.careeronestop.org/ CompetencyModel/pyramid.aspx?EHR=Y. Accessed December 5, 2011.

skills, education, or experience. To succeed, companies should develop core competencies or activities that a company performs better than its competition (Thompson, Strickland & Gamble, 2010). In a healthcare organization, competencies could focus both on clinical and administrative competencies. Therefore, the competency model provides an opportunity to assess existing competencies and any lack of competencies in different jobs. This analysis will be helpful when recruiting and selecting appropriate employees.

■ Job Design

As stated earlier, job analysis represents the building blocks of human resource management. Once job and workflow analyses have been performed, the next step is **job design,** which determines how the tasks, duties, and responsibilities will be performed and how the job fits into the organization. The focus of job design is to develop a strategy to maximize job efficiency, to promote health and safety in the work environment, and to encourage employee motivation (Noe, Hollenbeck, Gerhart & Wright, 2011). Job design can occur in healthcare organizations but can be difficult to implement because many jobs can only be performed by individuals with very specific job specifications such as nurses and physicians, who require specific licenses and maintain very specific skill sets (Fried & Fottler, 2008, p. 178).

Industrial engineering is the best way to analyze jobs to maximize efficiency. The American Institute of Industrial Engineers defines **industrial engineering** as the mathematical and natural science application to maximize labor efficiency utilizing appropriate equipment and task structure using time and motion studies. Once it determines the most efficient motions to perform a job, the organization recruits potential employees based on the skills needed to perform the job (Industrial Engineering, 2011). Although efficiency is important in healthcare operations, it is also important that a job design include a health and safety component. The Occupational Safety and Health Administration is responsible for implementing and enforcing labor regulations related to employee safety and health. **Ergonomics** is the study of the link between employees and their physical work environment to ensure that the conditions are optimal for employees to perform physically to the best of their abilities without causing undue stress on an employee's physical condition (Industrial Engineering, 2011). This is particularly true in the healthcare industry. Physical therapists are required to lift patients. Healthcare administrators may work long hours sitting at their desks. Surgeons perform arduous operations. All of these instances require equipment that is conducive to the employees providing the best performance possible; therefore equipment that is ergonomically designed has become more popular, which has resulted in a reduction of workplace injuries.

Based on the workflow analysis and job design, an organization defines a job with a written document that contains several components. The components typically include job identification, job responsibilities or functions, and job specifications. The **job identification** typically consists of the job title, the geographic location of the job, and the type of job—whether it is full time, management, or salaried. As discussed earlier, essential job functions are the primary duties of the position. Oftentimes, a job description may have a list of the **tasks, duties, and responsibilities** (**TDRs**) that are required. The **job specifications** identify the qualifications needed to be successful in the job, which consist of education, licensing, experience, and skills or competencies. These are often called **knowledge, skills, abilities, and other characteristics** (Mondy, 2012). Job conditions and any physical requirements are also indicated. Job applicants typically see a job posting, which provides many of those elements. A job posting is located on an organization's employment website, in a newspaper, or at a job fair. A job posting typically provides job identification, a job description, the minimum and preferred specifications for the job, and the list of job responsibilities.

▪ Job Redesign

The healthcare industry is a competitive industry, particularly in the nursing profession. There continues to be a shortage of nurses nationally. As a result, nurses have become disgruntled because their workload has increased resulting in the lowering of patient satisfaction and safety. A major task of job design is to redesign the structures of jobs to encourage and to motivate employees. Job enlargement, job rotation, and job enrichment are examples of **job redesign**. Job enrichment is the most common job redesign in the healthcare industry. **Job enlargement** broadens the types of tasks that are performed to make a job more interesting. It is considered a type of horizontal loading. For example, nurses may be given the responsibility of managing patients in several departments. **Job rotation** also increases job interest by transferring an employee from one job to another. It is a type of cross-training and provides variation to the employee. It is less common in health care because of licensing and accreditation issues with several types of jobs. **Job enrichment** increases the responsibility of the employee by increasing decision-making power within the employee's job. Job enrichment is a form of employee empowerment, providing more autonomy to the employee to encourage decision making and management skills. For example, a nurse may be asked to participate in strategic planning or in managing a quality improvement committee (Ozcan, 2009).

Other Types of Job Redesign

Self-Directed Work Teams

Many organizations, particularly healthcare organizations, organize employee teams to manage work goals. These teams are called **self-directed work teams**. Team members have control over the work schedule, and the employees are empowered to complete the work process as they design it. Healthcare organizations are inherently designed to produce work as a team. For example, the care of a patient with a chronic heart condition could comprise a team including the primary care provider, the specialist, the nurse, the pharmacist, and the physical therapist. They all collaborate to achieve their ultimate goal of providing quality care to their patient. Healthcare studies indicate that high teamwork performance is the result of commitment to collaboration, commitment to quality outcome, and commitment to the organization. This is achieved by ensuring strong communication in the organization so that employees are clear about the organizational goals (Leggat, 2007).

Depending on the job position in the organization, different training may be required to ensure a high-performance team. For example, many clinicians also have their own practices, so training must be provided to ensure that the employees have a commitment to the organization where they treat their patients. Entry-level positions in a team may require different training than that for a middle manager in a team concept because the focus of these positions is different. Entry-level positions are less focused on management than are middle manager positions. Senior management focuses more on organizational goal completion rather than on task completion. Although teams are evident in many aspects of health care, training needs to be customized to ensure a quality outcome (Wallick & Stager, 2001).

Job Sharing

Job sharing occurs when two employees share the same position. This is an attractive option for employees who are valuable but want more time for personal obligations. It is becoming more popular in health care. A 2010 survey indicated that healthcare organizations were going to offer more opportunities for job sharing (Careerbuilder.com, 2010).

Flexible Work Schedules

Flexible work schedules provide flexibility in a work schedule. This option is an attractive choice for employees. **Flextime** allows employees to start and end their workdays at alternative times within specified guidelines. Employees may need different work schedules for family obligations, for example. Healthcare surveys indicate that nearly 75% of healthcare employers would offer flexible work schedules as a benefit. Approximately 10% of employers are also considering summer work hours (Colonna, 2005). This can be motivating to employees but also can be a service to the organization because healthcare consumers often require 24-hour attention.

Telework

Healthcare organizations recognize that technology continues to play a vital role in healthcare delivery. **Telework,** or telecommuting in an organization, designates certain employees to work outside the physical organization. Telework is becoming more common in the healthcare industry, as clinicians are providing more care to their patients via telemedicine. For example, SSM Health care, which won the Malcolm Baldridge National Quality Award and owns, manages, and is affiliated with 20 acute care hospitals, developed a telework contact center to deliver care. The SSM Health care telework contact center served as the benchmark for the industry by establishing a telework center where employees would be on call for all healthcare needs. Results indicate that operating expenses were lowered and employee satisfaction was increased. More nurses were attracted to working at SSM Health Care because of this telework opportunity (Healthlinesystems.com, 2011).

■ Conclusion

Evaluating the workflow of any organization is the first step to developing jobs for individuals to perform that will ensure the workflow produces the desired outputs of the organization. Once the workflow is analyzed, the next step is to create jobs for individuals who will be employed by the organization and be responsible for producing the output of the organization. Prior to creating a job, a job analysis must be performed to determine which types of activities will be performed within a certain position in the organization. Job analysis is the foundation of human resource management because the analysis of a job is required before an organization begins to recruit individuals for specific jobs. At the conclusion of a job analysis, a written job description and written job specifications are developed that outline the responsibilities, skills, and experience needed to perform the job successfully.

An important component of job development is how jobs are designed so that the health and safety of employees are ensured through ergonomics, the work is efficiently performed, and employees are motivated to perform at a high level. Motivational job designs include flextime; job sharing; job enlargement, enrichment, and rotation; and telework. The same process must be performed if the organization decides to alter the way a service is being offered. For example, if electronic medical records will be implemented in a healthcare facility, it is necessary to determine the current workflow patterns and then redesign the projected workflow to accommodate the new technology. If an organization is diligent in these processes of job analysis and design, it will help the organization perform at its highest level.

■ Vocabulary

Academic competencies
Competencies
Competency model
Element
Ergonomics
Essential job functions
Flexible work schedules
Flextime
Industrial engineering
Inputs
Job
Job analysis
Job analyst
Job design

Job enlargement
Job enrichment
Job identification
Job redesign
Job rotation
Job sharing
Job specifications
Knowledge, skills, abilities, and
    other characteristics
Management Position Description
    Questionnaire
Micromotion
Occupational Information Network
    (O*NET)

Outputs
Personal effectiveness competencies
Position Analysis Questionnaire
Self-directed work teams
Task
Tasks, duties, and responsibilities

Telework
Work activity
Workflow
Workflow analysis
Workplace competencies

■ References

About DOL (2011). Available at: http://www.dol.gov/dol/aboutdol/main.htm. Accessed December 11, 2011.

ASU PAQ [Position Analysis Questionnaire] (2008). Available at: http://www.asu.edu/hr/documents/PAQuestionnaire.pdf. Accessed January 5, 2011.

Building Blocks Model (2010). Available at: http://www.careeronestop.org/CompetencyModel/pyramid.aspx. Accessed January 4, 2011.

Byars, L. & Rue, L. (2006). *Human Resource Management* (8th ed.). New York, NY: McGraw-Hill/Irwin, p. 64.

Careerbuilder.com (2010). One in Five Health Care Employers Plan to Hire in 2010. Available at: http://www.careerbuilder.com/aboutus/pressreleasesdetail.aspx?id=pr549&sd=1/27/2010. Accessed January 9, 2011.

Colonna, J. (2005). Why Teams Matter in Healthcare: Seven Characteristics That Define Successful Teams. Available at: http://findarticles.com/p/articles/mi_m0BPC/is_7_29. Accessed January 9, 2011.

Essex, D. (2000). The many layers of workflow automation. *Healthcare Informatics*, June:128–135.

Fried, B. & Fottler, M, (2008). *Human Resources in Health Care* (3rd ed.). Chicago: Health Administration Press: p. 178.

Healthlinesystems.com (2011). Sip Coffee While in Your Slippers: How to Succeed with Agents at Home. Available at: http://www.healthlinesystems.com/hottopics_021605.aspx. Accessed January 9, 2011.

How Do I Perform a Detailed Work Analysis? (2011). Available at: http://www.hrsa.gov/healthit/toolbox/HealthITAdoptiontoolbox/SystemImplementation/workflowanalysis.html. Accessed December 11, 2011.

Human Resources (2011). Training and Labor Relations Manager and Specialists. Job Analysts. Available at: http://www.bls.gov/oco/ocos021.htm. Accessed January 8, 2011.

Industrial Engineering (2011). Available at: http://www.iienet2.org/Details.aspx?id=1848. Accessed January 9, 2011.

Leggat, S. (2007). Defining teamwork competencies. *BMC Health Services Research*, 7(17).

Mathis, R. & Jackson, J. (2006a). *Human Resource Management* (11th ed.). Mason, OH: Thomson/South-Western, pp. 175–189.

Mathis, R. & Jackson, J. (2006b). *Human Resource Management* (11th ed.). Mason, OH: Thomson/South-Western, p. 179.

Mathis, R. & Jackson, J. (2006c). *Human Resource Management* (11th ed.). Mason, OH: Thomson/South-Western, pp. 107–108.

Mondy, R. (2012). *Human Resource Management*. Upper Saddle River, NJ: Prentice Hall: pp. 87–88.

Noe, R., Hollenbeck, J., Gerhart B. & Wright, P. (2012). *Fundamentals of Human Resource Management* (3rd ed.). McGraw-Hill/Irwin, pp. 29–30.

O*NET (2011). Available at: http://online.onetcenter.org/. Accessed January 5, 2011.

Ozcan, Y. (2009). *Quantitative Methods in Healthcare Management* (2nd ed.). San Francisco, CA: Jossey-Bass, pp. 120–130.

Thompson, A., Strickland, A. & Gamble, J. (2010). *Crafting and Executing Strategy: Concepts and Cases* (17th ed.). Boston, MA: McGraw-Hill/Irwin, pp. 108–110.

Wallick, W. & Stager, K. (2001). Healthcare managers' roles, competencies and outputs in organizational performance improvement/practitioner response. *Journal of Healthcare Management,* 47(6):390–402.

What Is NAICS? (2010). Available at: http://www.bls.gov/sae/saewhatis.htm. Accessed July 11, 2010.

STUDENT WORKBOOK ACTIVITY 3.1

Complete the following case scenarios based on the information provided in the chapter. Your answer must be *in your own words*.

Real-Life Applications: Case Scenario 1

As an HR consultant, you have been asked to perform a job analysis for a local hospital. It is a complex job, and you need some tools to help with the analysis.

Activity

Select two tools that you believe would be helpful and describe why they would be useful for your consulting project.

Responses

_____

_____

_____

_____

_____

Real-Life Applications: Case Scenario 2

You are working toward your master's degree in human resource management. One of your assignments is to write job descriptions and job specifications for different healthcare positions.

Activity

Choose two healthcare positions and, based on the tools discussed in the chapter, write up the two healthcare positions.

Responses

_____

_____

_____

_____

_____

Real-Life Applications: Case Scenario 3

Defining competencies in an organization is important to the strategic management of an organization.

Activity

Discuss the competency model as it relates to your organization. If you are not currently working, select an organization where you would like to work. Select three competencies of your organization that you can apply to the model.

Responses

_____

_____

_____

_____

_____

Real-Life Applications: Case Scenario 4

Workflow analysis is an integral component of any organization. You would like to start a home healthcare agency and believe you need to perform a workflow analysis to determine what type of workflow will occur in your organization.

Activity

Using the Internet to research home health agency staffing and work activities and using the workflow analysis model, prepare a workflow analysis of your new business.

Responses

_____

_____

_____

_____

_____

STUDENT WORKBOOK ACTIVITY 3.2

In Your Own Words

Please describe the following core concepts in your own words.

Job enlargement:

_____

_____

_____

_____

Essential job functions:

_____

_____

_____

_____

Industrial engineering:

_____

_____

_____

_____

Ergonomics:

_____

_____

_____

_____

Telework:

_____

_____

_____

_____

Job sharing:

_____

_____

_____

_____

Job analyst:

_____

_____

_____

_____

Position Analysis Questionnaire:

_____

_____

_____

_____

Workflow analysis:

_____

_____

_____

_____

O*NET:

_____

_____

_____

_____

STUDENT WORKBOOK ACTIVITY 3.3

Internet Exercises

Write your answers in the spaces provided.

- Visit each of the websites listed in the text that follows.
- Name the organization.
- Locate its mission statement on its website. If the organization does not have a mission statement, describe its purpose.

- Provide a brief overview of the activities of the organization.
- Apply this organization to the chapter information.

Websites
http://www.healthit.ahrq.gov
Organization name:

_____

Mission statement:

_____

_____

_____

Overview of activities:

_____

_____

_____

Application to chapter information:

_____

_____

_____

http://onlineonetcenter.org
Organization name:

_____

Mission statement:

_____

_____

_____

Overview of activities:

_____

_____

_____

Application to chapter information:

_____

_____

_____

http://www.bls.gov
Organization name:

_____

Mission statement:

_____

_____

_____

Overview of activities:

_____

_____

_____

Application to chapter information:

_____

_____

_____

http://www.careerbuilder.com

Organization name:

_____

Mission statement:

_____

_____

_____

Overview of activities:

_____

_____

_____

Application to chapter information:

_____

_____

_____

http://www.healthlinesystem.com

Organization name:

_____

Mission statement:

_____

_____

_____

Overview of activities:

_____

_____

_____

Application to chapter information:

_____

_____

_____

http://www.dol.gov

Organization name:

_____

Mission statement:

_____

_____

_____

Overview of activities:

_____

_____

_____

Application to chapter information:

_____

_____

_____

STUDENT ACTIVITY 3.4: DISCUSSION BOARDS FOR ONLINE, HYBRID, AND TRADITIONAL CLASSES

Discussion Board Guidelines

The discussion board is used in online and web-enhanced courses in place of classroom lectures and discussion. The board can also be used as an enhancement to traditional classes. The discussion board is the way in which the students "link together" as a class. The following are guidelines to help focus on the discussion topic and to define the roles and responsibilities of the discussion coordinator and other members of the class. The educator will be the discussion moderator for this course.

1. The educator will post the discussion topic and directions for the upcoming week. These postings should all be responses to the original topic or in responses to other students' responses. When people respond to what someone else has posted, they should start the posting with the person's name so it is clear which message they are responding to. **A response such as "Yes" or "I agree" does**

not count for credit. Your responses must be in your own words. You cannot copy and paste from the text.

2. Postings (especially responses) should include enough information so the message is clear but should not be so long that it becomes difficult to follow. Remember, this is like talking to someone in a classroom setting. The postings should reflect the content of the text or other assignments. If you retrieve information from the Internet, the hyperlink must be cited.

3. Students should check the discussion daily to see if new information has been posted that requires their attention and response.

Good discussion will often include different points of view. Students should feel free to disagree or "challenge" others to support their positions or ideas. All discussions must be handled in a respectful manner. The following are discussion boards for this chapter.

Discussion Boards

1. Describe the competency model. Do you think this is a good way to analyze the skills needed to perform in health care? Develop a model for a hospice care center and post.

2. Of the building blocks of the competency model, which competency level is the most important and why?

3. What is the difference between a job description and a job specification? Research using the Internet and develop a job description and job specifications of a healthcare job.

4. What is the purpose of job redesign? Which job redesign described in the text would appeal to you and why?

Recruiting a Healthcare Workforce

DID YOU KNOW THAT?

- An indirect method of employee recruitment is a company presence on social media websites.
- More healthcare organizations are using shadowing programs as a recruitment method, which allow a potential employee to follow an existing employee for a day.
- The Health on the Net Foundation was created in 1995 to ensure that healthcare organizations provide reliable information on the Internet.
- The employee selection process must be legally defensible, which means the process must be objective and fair to all applicants.
- A bona fide occupational qualification means that a particular characteristic of an individual allows an organization to discriminate against protected individuals.

■ Introduction

Recruitment is an organizational process of attracting applicants for job openings in an organization. Selection of the appropriate candidates occurs from a pool of qualified applicants (Byars & Rue, 2006). The main goal of the recruitment process is to generate a qualified pool of applicants to select from to support the success of an organization. For the recruitment process to be successful, it is important that the recruiters use job analysis to develop appropriate job openings to attract qualified applicants (Fried & Fottler, 2008). The next step is to select the best potential candidates for the organization. The recruitment and selection processes are priorities of any organization. This chapter will describe the steps in successful recruitment in healthcare organizations, the sources of recruitment, successful recruiter characteristics, a legal selection process, and the importance of hiring a diverse workforce.

■ Recruitment Methods

Organizations recruit both internally and externally. Internally, organizations recruit in three ways. First, organizations ask current employees for referrals. Most referrals will be quality referrals because a poor referral will reflect poorly on the employee. If the referral is successful, the organization may reward the employee for the successful referral. Second, management will promote from within the organization. Organizations like to reward quality employees with a promotion or transfer to a new job. This can be an advantage to the organization because the employee is already familiar with the organization and is a known entity to the organization. Promoting from within is an incentive for all employees to work harder. **Internal recruitment** is also less expensive and less time consuming. The only potential disadvantage of internal hiring is when an organization is changing its organizational culture or strategic plan. It could be a disadvantage to promote an existing employee, as she or he may have an established organizational mindset.

Third, an organization will hire from its internship program. Many organizations offer either paid or unpaid internships, which are often a 6- to 12-month position in an organization usually staffed by graduate and undergraduate college students. Internship programs are typically a partnership between an organization and an educational institution where the student works part-time and receives educational credit for the work. The partnership agrees upon designated work activities for the student. It gives the student an opportunity to experience healthcare working conditions and provides him or her a glimpse into "real-life" experiences. It also provides an opportunity to observe whether the student would be a good employee for the organization. Some universities require students to complete an internship as part of their graduation requirement (Dessler, 2012).

External recruitment can be obtained from many different sources. **Advertising** in designated publications (print media) has been common for decades. Targeting of clinical publications for nurses and physicians, for example, is a common way to recruit. However, what has become more common is **job postings** placed on an organization's website. It is less expensive and can capture a larger population. However, the downside of electronic job postings is that a posting can generate hundreds of unqualified applicants. In addition to placing a job posting on the organization's website, the organization will also place an electronic posting on a career website. For example, the career site http://www.gohealthcarejobs.org has postings for healthcare jobs nationally.

Government Sources

Local, state, and federal government employment departments are used when recruiting for government openings. They post positions on their websites for both external and internal openings. The websites for federal government openings are http://federaljobs .net/federal_jobs_opening.htm and http://www.usajobs.gov. Local government agencies also use local information cable channels to broadcast openings in the local area.

In 2001, Children's Hospital in Boston implemented a **shadowing program** to recruit nurses from hospitals. The organization advertises the program in the local newspaper or online, asking if any nurses are interested in following a nurse employee for a day while the nurse employee is performing a typical daily work routine. Nurses who visit also meet with the management of the surgical program to learn about the program. This also provides an opportunity for the hospital to assess the visiting nurses in a clinical setting (Shermont & Murphy, 2006).

Private Employment Agencies

Organizations use private employment agencies to recruit both senior-level and lower-level employees. Agencies often charge an expensive fee for their services, but they are responsible for the entire process and typically generate very qualified applicants.

Temporary Employee Services

Temporary employee agencies provide employees for short-term and long-term assignments in all industries. They charge a company a designated wage for the employee and are responsible for paying the temporary employee's wages. The **temporary employment agency** often provides employee benefits. For example, Maxim Healthcare Solutions, established in 1988 because of the continued nursing shortage, is the largest private employment agency nationally. It places qualified medical personnel for both temporary and permanent assignments (About Maxim, 2011). When a company like Maxim Healthcare Solutions places a short-term employee in a healthcare organization, it provides an opportunity for the company to observe the employee to assess his or her work ethic and to determine if the employee would fit in the organization.

Educational Recruitment Activities: Job Fairs

Many healthcare organizations will hold job fairs at educational institutions that have healthcare programs. The company recruiters will ask for graduating students' résumés and will conduct interviews at the job fair. They may also ask students to sign up so the job recruiters can decide prior to the event exactly who should receive an interview.

■ Direct and Indirect External Recruitment Methods

There are **direct methods of recruiting**, which consist of an organization actively searching for candidates for specific job openings. There are also **indirect methods of recruiting** such as establishment of a **social media** presence (Byars & Rue, 2006). Historically, organizations would place job openings in newspapers and trade publications, which were often expensive. Electronic job recruiting is more common because it is cost effective.

Many organizations post their job openings on their websites for public viewing. It is one of the most inexpensive ways to post jobs. Organizations may also post jobs for internal application only, meaning that only existing employees can apply. In addition to company recruitment, **electronic job recruitment** occurs on general career websites such as Monster.com and careerbuilder.com. Many healthcare recruiting sites focus on certain healthcare jobs such as nurse, physician, and chiropractor. The following are only a few examples of the diverse opportunities for electronic job recruitment:

- http://www.nationalmedicalsearch.com: A national search agency that recruits physicians and nurses.
- http://www.foundationmedicalstaffing.com: Recruits specifically for the dialysis industry.
- http://www.soliant.com: Recruits for specialty professionals nationally.
- http://www.ihrcanada.com: Recruits healthcare professionals for the Middle East.

Electronic Job Fairs

The electronic job fair is a newer method of job recruitment. Electronic job fairs are similar to traditional job fairs because they have a designated target and city and designated dates with specific hours for the contact. Typically, employers are charged a fee for participating in the electronic job fair, but the fees are approximately one third the cost of a traditional job fair because the electronic job fair eliminates travel and setup costs (ejobfairs.net, 2011). The job seeker pays no fee. The job seeker signs up on the website, uploads his or her résumé, creates a generic introduction, and then searches for electronic job fairs. Employees contact company recruiters directly and interview electronically. Users can follow, for instance, ejobfairs.net on Twitter.

Social Media

An indirect method of recruitment is the presence of healthcare organizations on Facebook, Twitter, and LinkedIn. The Cleveland Clinic, which is one of the most highly regarded healthcare systems worldwide, is progressive in its use of electronic media to recruit potential employees. On its home page, there are links to social media outlets and a link to careers at Cleveland Clinic (http://www.clevelandclinic .org). Its Facebook page promotes the organization and educates consumers about their health. Its LinkedIn page focuses on past and present employees of the clinic, which gives them an opportunity to network with each other. Its Twitter home page has links to the Centers for Disease Control and Prevention and to other government agencies that focus on health issues. The Cleveland Clinic is marketing itself via these electronic venues.

Health on the Net Foundation

Created in 1995, the **Health on the Net Foundation (HON)** is a watchdog of online health organizations. The Economic and Social Council of the United Nations accredits this non-governmental organization, which focuses on ensuring that healthcare information is reliable. The foundation's HON Code of Conduct certifies that an organization's website complies with eight principles, which are as follows:

1. Information is provided by qualified authors.
2. Information supports but does not replace the doctor–patient relationship.
3. The confidentiality of website users and visitors is maintained.
4. Information is sourced.
5. The site supports any performance claims.
6. Contact information is available.
7. Funding sources are identified.
8. Advertising policy is clear.

The foundation also has HONsearches, HONtools, and HONtopics—all guaranteed by HON to be correct (HON Code of Conduct, 2011). This type of certification is another way of marketing an organization. HON has certified the Cleveland Clinic. It demonstrates the quality of the Cleveland Clinic. Job seekers are attracted to an organization that supports ethical behavior.

■ Successful Recruiters

Recruiters are designated employees or human resources (HR) specialists who are responsible for attracting the best employees to their organizations. They are considered to be the face of an organization, and it is important to select the appropriate employees to recruit new employees. Although many recruiters work in an HR department, research indicates that candidates prefer to be interviewed by employees who work in different departments in an organization, although assembling a team of recruiters that includes an HR specialist who is familiar with HR policies and procedures may be an option (Noe, Hollenbeck, Gerhart & Wright, 2012a).

Michael Homula (2005) stated there are several characteristics that successful recruiters possess including excellent oral communication skills, the ability to develop a rapport with the candidates, the ability to be a good listener, loyalty to the organization, the ability to interpret the nonverbal behavior of candidates, understanding of the organizational culture, and dedication to recruiting the best possible candidates for the organization. It is important for an organization carefully to select the best employees for this type of activity and to provide training, if necessary, on successful recruitment methods.

■ Recruitment Evaluations: Source Yield Ratios

There are many employee recruitment methods used in the healthcare industry. Print media include trade magazines, social media, company websites, career fairs, and employment agencies. A company will analyze which of the methods produces the greatest number of qualified employees to interview and consequently hire. **Source yield ratios,** calculated as percentages, evaluate the type of recruitment activity that ultimately produces a candidate that accepts a position with the company. For example, a company will calculate a source yield ratio for external recruitment methods such as advertising in a trade magazine or using the Internet. The source yield ratio can also be calculated for internal recruitment methods such as employee referrals or internal job postings. Tables 4.1 and 4.2 indicate the source yield calculations for both external and internal recruitment methods. Table 4.1 reveals that advertising in the trade magazine and on the website produce a source yield of 10% and 20%, respectively. Table 4.2 outlines the calculations for internal recruitment of employee referrals and internal job postings, which produce a higher source yield ratio of 50%. Each step in the process could also be calculated using the source yield ratio. Of the number of applicants, a source yield ratio could be calculated for number of interviews accepted, the number of applicants who receive offers, and the number of new hires. A higher percentage indicates the method is an effective way of finding new hires (Source Yield, 2011).

Table 4.1 Source Yield Ratio Examples: External Recruitment

	Trade Magazine	Internet Website
No. of applicants	100	1000
No. of hires	10	200
Calculation	10/100	200/1000
Source Yield Ratio	10%	20%

Table 4.2 Source Yield Ratio Examples: Internal Recruitment

	Internal Job Postings	Employee Referrals
No. of applicants	50	20
No. of hires	25	10
Calculation	25/50	10/20
Source Yield Ratio	50%	50%

In addition to the source yield ratio analysis, the cost of each recruitment process must also be analyzed. Budgeting is always a concern for recruitment. If the company were recruiting for a senior management position, it would most likely spend more money on the recruitment and hiring process. If the recruitment were targeting lower-level positions, then the company would likely spend less on the recruitment process, which is not always the most prudent decision, particularly in health care. There is so much teamwork involved in health care that employees at all levels in a healthcare organization play a role in patient care, and therefore it is important to place a priority on recruitment at all levels.

Typically, the most expensive recruitment method is using an employment agency, and the least expensive is electronic job posting because this is often a feature of a company's website. The company may decide to pay a fee, which varies, to post an opening on a career website. The organization must track the recruiting expenses of a position and calculate how many candidates were hired. Another factor in determining the success of any recruitment process is the time required to complete a process successfully. In a recent survey, it was determined that employment agencies often take 30 days to hire and the Internet took only 12 days, so time also needs to be factored into the evaluation process (Mathis & Jackson, 2006).

■ Selection Process

The **selection process** consists of choosing the best individuals for an organization. The recruitment process is implemented to find the best employee. There is a strong linkage between recruiting and selecting. If there is a poor recruitment strategy, there will not be a qualified pool of applicants for selection. As with any human resource management process, there should be collaboration between the HR department and the managers of the organization. Once the recruitment process is completed, the organization will have a pool of applicant résumés to review. A generic selection process consists of (1) initial screening of the applications, (2) interviewing qualified applicants, (3) administering any tests, (4) conducting a reference and background check, and (5) offering a job to the best individual (Dessler, 2012). If an organization has a designated HR department, then there will be an initial screening of the résumés by HR to determine which candidates are qualified. If there is no HR department, there will be a designated individual or committee to screen the applications. To ensure reliability and validity in the process, organizations use a résumé rating tool for candidates' résumés. The tool provides a standardization of the résumé evaluation process.

Based on the job description and job specifications, a tool, either electronic or manual, is developed. All applicant résumés are rated to determine if applicants meet the specifications of the job and if they have the skills to perform the job. In some organizations, there will be a telephone interview as part of the screening process. Once the résumés are initially screened for qualifications, then telephone or video-conferencing interviews may occur to screen the candidates prior to inviting the top prospects for a face-to-face interview.

Types of Selection Tests

As part of the selection process, different tests will be administered to applicants. **Physical ability tests** focus on strength and endurance such as that for carrying and lifting of equipment. **Psychomotor tests** measure a person's hand–eye coordination. **Aptitude tests** may be given to assess a candidate's ability to perform a certain task such as laboratory analysis or reading X-rays. There is also a **healthcare aptitude test**, which analyzes the ability of individuals to be compassionate with patients and their ability to work with teams (employtest.com, 2011). **Cognitive ability tests** measure memory, critical thinking, and verbal and math comprehension, which applied to an organization includes problem solving, planning and organizing, and reasoning. Research indicates that these tests can accurately predict job performance (Arnold, 2011).

Rather than implementing individual selection tests, **identity (attitude and aptitude) tests** have been developed that assess not only cognitive ability but also risk profiles for drug use and workplace violence, service and helping orientation, team player potential, trustworthiness and reliability, workplace skills, and workplace personality, and these tests can be customized for the healthcare industry (totaltesting.com, 2011).

Personality tests assess an applicant's characteristics that could affect the work environment. The test scores are based on 100% with an average score of 50%; therefore a score of 70% would indicate a higher demonstration of a particular personality trait. Personality experts have developed a set of personality traits that demonstrate different levels of performance in the workplace in different job positions. These **Big Five Personality Traits** include extraversion, conscientiousness, agreeableness, emotional stability, and openness to experience. **Extraversion** refers to the degree an employee is open and outgoing and is energized by relationships with other employees. Applicants who score high on this test would more likely perform better in sales, management, and teamwork. Those who did not score high may be more suited for research positions, which have less interaction with other employees. **Conscientiousness** measures how goal oriented an individual is and if he or she is disciplined in the workplace. These types of employees are an asset to any organization and are very suitable for teamwork. **Agreeableness** measures an employee's sensitivity to other employees, whether he or she succumbs to peer pressure, is willing to help others, and has a positive attitude toward others. These types of employees work well in team situations. An applicant who scores high on **emotional stability** indicates a high tolerance for stressful situations and heavy work demands. Such individuals perform well in different industries including health care with its stressful environment. **Openness to experience** indicates an applicant's preference for a variety of responsibilities in his or her job description. Such individuals would perform well in a job redesign such as job enrichment or job enlargement. They tend to be very imaginative and are sensitive to the emotions of others. Applicants who score high and low on this trait tend to perform well in teams; however, those who score high on this trait tend to ignore rules (Hitt, Miller & Colella, 2006). Lievens, Coetsier, Fruyt, and De Maeseneer (2002) performed personality tests on 800 premedical students studying at five universities, and the results indicated that students who scored high on their clinical exams also scored high on extraversion and agreeableness. Medical students who scored low on conscientiousness and openness to experience scored poorly on clinical exams. Lievens and colleagues' conclusions indicated that the test results were indicative of medical students' performance in the medical field.

The Big Five Personality Traits could also be used as a basis for developing interview questions to assess the type personality of the candidate. For example, if the interviewers would like to investigate the conscientiousness of a candidate, the questions would focus on whether the candidate likes to be prepared for a situation, if he or she pays attention to details, accomplishes tasks immediately, likes order, and is precise in his or her work. If the interviewer were interested in emotional stability, the questions would focus on mood swings and reaction to pressure. Openness to experience questions would probe if the candidate is imaginative, is creative, and follows rules and regulations. Agreeableness characteristics could be revealed by asking questions about empathy, making people feel comfortable, and compassion. Although a company could perform a valid and reliable Big Five Personality test, asking interview questions that focus on these characteristics as well would support any personality test results.

Honesty Tests

Many companies are now using **honesty or integrity tests** with applicants, although there have been questions about the validity of these tests because applicants can fake honesty on the tests. Companies use these tests as a statement to applicants that dishonesty is not tolerated in the organization. Because their validity has been questioned, it is important for these tests to be only one component of the whole process (Mathis & Jackson, 2006).

Background Checks

Background checks consist of verifying information on the applicant's résumé, asking for academic transcripts, speaking with those given as references, and running a credit check. The applicant is told that a background check will be performed. An in-depth background check or **criminal background check** may also be performed to assess any past criminal offenses. The applicant must acknowledge in writing that a criminal check will be performed. More companies are performing a criminal background check because if an individual is hired and acts illegally or hurts another employee, the company could be held liable for not providing a safe working environment. The author has been involved in hiring processes where the candidate has withdrawn from the process because he or she learned that a criminal background check would be performed; thus, these checks can be a deterrent for applicants that may not be suitable for an organization. Although most companies require references from former employers, some former employers have been sued for providing a poor reference, so many former employers now only provide general information about when a former employee worked for the organization and his or her position and responsibilities (Mathis & Jackson, 2006).

■ Interviewing Candidates

Once the screening occurs, a list will be prepared of candidates to be invited to an interview. Usually, the employees of the department needing the new employee will participate in the interview. If the organization has an HR department, the interviewers will be trained by HR. Interviews can be held by individuals or by a panel. The interviews can be face to face or by telephone or another electronic method. Interviewers can ask very structured or unstructured questions. Regardless of the type of interview, it is important that there is validity and reliability in the process.

Types of Interviews

Structured interviews are standardized questions that all interviewees must answer. Standardized questions allow a comparison between the candidates. The questions are prepared in advance. A **situational interview** is a type of structured interview that consists of structured questions that focus on how the applicant would behave in certain situations. An example of a question in a situational interview for a nurse candidate is the following: "If your shift replacement, who is the daughter of the nurse manager, was consistently tardy, how would you handle the situation?" A **behavioral interview** is similar but focuses on how the candidate handled a situation in his or her past. An example of a behavioral question would be the following: "Describe your behavior when you had to deal with a difficult patient." Structured interviews are more reliable and valid because there is standardization (Byars & Rue, 2006). **Unstructured**

Table 4.3 Common Interview Questions

What are your strengths and weaknesses?

How can you contribute to the success of this organization?

Why do you want to work for us?

Describe a situation that you were in within the past 2 years that demonstrated your leadership.

Have you ever had to discipline someone? Describe the situation.

If your boss asked you to do something that may be illegal, what would you do?

What skills do you have that would contribute to the success of this job?

Define ethics in your own words.

Why did you decide to choose health care as your career?

Why are you leaving your current job?

---

interviews consist of the interviewer asking the applicant questions based on answers to previous questions. There is less preparation for this type of interview. Although the interviewer may obtain valuable information about the applicant, it is difficult to compare applicants for the same position using this type of interview. Table 4.3 lists some typical questions the author has commonly asked candidates.

■ Validity and Reliability of the Employment Process

Every component of the employment process must be job related to avoid any issues of discrimination. To ensure that a step in the process is objective, it is important to assess the validity and reliability of the step. The term **validity** is a statistical term that refers to the extent a measurement such as a test actually measures what it says it measures. **Reliability** is a statistical term that refers to the extent that the same measurement such as a test repeatedly measures the same characteristic if the test is given multiple times to different individuals. For example, valid and reliable employment tests such as selection tests must evaluate the actual skill or trait repeatedly regardless of who is taking the test (Mondy, 2012).

Content and Criterion Validity

Content validity is developed when a selection tool evaluates skills or knowledge that is used in a job application. For example, X-ray technician applicants may be asked about how to take an X-ray or a nursing applicant may be asked about how to take blood from a patient. The test will ask questions related specifically to activities related to a job. A selection tool must also have **criterion-validity**, which means that the scores on a test will be related to job performance predictions. If applicants score poorly on a test, they most likely will not perform well on their jobs, and if they score high on their test, their job performance will be high (Dessler, 2012).

Once a candidate is hired, the selection tool's results will be compared with the actual job performance. The comparison will be measured by a correlation test, which examines the relationship between two factors such as test results and job performance. **Correlation coefficients** always range from –1 to +1. The sign of the correlation coefficient (+ , –) defines the direction of the relationship, either positive or negative.

Taking the positive aspect of a coefficient relationship, a correlation coefficient of 50% or less indicates a low correlation; 51% to 79% indicates a low to moderate correlation; 80% to 89% indicates moderate to strong connections between two factors; and greater than 90% indicates a very high correlation between two factors. Therefore, a higher percentage score for the selection test and job performance correlation indicates the selection tool should be used.

■ Legal Ramifications of the Selection Process

The selection process must be **legally defensible,** which means the process must be objective and fair to all applicants (Noe, Hollenbeck, Gerhart & Wright, 2012b). The Equal Employment Opportunity Commission (EEOC) is the federal commission that monitors and enforces labor regulations to ensure that the employment process is non-discriminatory, which means that every component of the process must be objective and that no protected-class individual who is qualified is excluded from the process because of a flawed step. Therefore, all solicited résumés that are submitted for a job opening must be reviewed objectively to ensure there are no biases in the process. Protected-class applicants may question why they did not receive an interview if they felt they were qualified for the job. If the selection process is rigorously maintained with documentation at all steps of the process, the company and the employees will be protected. Table 4.4 is a job interview rubric to assess each candidate's performance. This supports the legally defensible process of selection. Using a standardized tool such as the rubric enables the interviewers to compare the performances of the various candidates for a position.

■ Characteristics of Good Interviewers

Similar to the recruitment process, the use of effective interviewers is very important to attract high-quality candidates to accept positions with an organization. Like the recruiters, it is important that the interviewers receive training to ensure they ask the appropriate questions and are comfortable with developing a rapport with the

Table 4.4 Job Interview Assessment Rubric

Candidate's Name: _____ Date: _____

Time of Interview: _____ Time Arrived: _____

Job Opening: _____ Interviewer: _____

Action Observed	Unacceptable Action (0 points)	Improvement Needed (5 points)	Acceptable Action (10 points)
Interview preparation	Late for interview, does not shake hands, no résumé or references.	Shows up on time, doesn't shake hands, résumé but no references.	Shows up early, shakes hands, has résumé and references.
Organizational interest	Knows nothing about the company or makes up information.	Knows some general information about the company.	Has researched the company thoroughly, which is apparent by answers given.
Job interest	Asks no questions about job.	Asks one or two questions about job.	Asks three or more questions about job.
Personal appearance	Dressed very inappropriately (too much makeup, jewelry, cologne, sandals, shorts, T-shirt). Unkempt appearance.	Dressed inappropriately No professional dress. Dressed in casual clothing. Neat appearance.	Dressed in appropriate attire; professional appearance. No sandals, tennis shoes, T-shirt, shorts, short skirt, Neat appearance.
Interview responses	Answers with "yes" or "no" and fails to elaborate. No eye contact. Appears nervous.	Gives well-constructed responses, but sounds rehearsed. Minimal eye contact.	Gives well-constructed, responses that seem genuine. Good eye contact. Confident.
Column Scores:____	Total Column____	Total Column____	Total Column:____
			Total Score of all Columns:

applicants to encourage quality responses. It is also important that the interviewer be prepared. The interviewers should review all résumés so that they are familiar with each candidate. Using a résumé review tool is an excellent method of providing inter-rater reliability of the reviewers. Table 4.5 and Table 4.6 provide an example of a tool that

Table 4.5 Example of a Job Posting

HEALTHCARE INFORMATION TECHNOLOGY DIRECTOR

JOB IDENTIFICATION:

Company: Health Is Yours Hospital

Location: Lady Lake, FL 32159

Job Type: Full-Time Title: Healthcare Information Technology Director

JOB DESCRIPTION: Implementation of an electronic health record system for a large hospital.

MINIMUM JOB SPECIFICATIONS FOR POSITION:
- Master of Science in Healthcare Informatics.
- 5 years of experience in IT management in a hospital setting.

JOB RESPONSIBILITIES:
- Manage the evaluation process of current patient system for electronic data system transfer.
- Make recommendations to senior management regarding electronic health record software.
- Develop training program for clinical staff for EHR software.
- Direct supervision of 10 IT staff.
- Implement new EHR system.

PREFERRED JOB SPECIFICATIONS:
- 10 years of management experience in hospital data systems.
- 5 years of supervisory experience.
- 2 years of experience with EHR systems implementation.
- Ability to manage a complex IT system using analytic and problem-solving skills.
- Excellent oral and written communication skills.

Please submit cover letter, résumé, and three references to:
http://www.HealthisYours.org/careers/InformationTechnolgyDirector
Any questions: Call the HR Department at 864-555-2000 or e-mail hrm@ healthisyours.com

Table 4.6 Résumé Evaluation Tool: Information Technology Director

Applicant Name _____

PART I: Screening of Minimum Qualifications – Indicated in Job Posting

1. Minimum education level for position: Master of   Yes __   No __
   Science Healthcare Informatics

   Other_____   Yes__   No__

2. Five years of experience in hospital IT setting   Yes__   No__

Signature of Screening Reviewer _____ Date _____

If applicant does not meet minimum position qualifications, do not proceed to Part II.

PART II: Preferred Qualifications Review – Indicated in Job Posting

• 10 years of hospital data management	Yes	No
• 5 years of supervisory experience	Yes	No
Comments:	___ no. of years	
• 2 years of EHR system implementation	Yes	No
Comments:	___ no. of years	
• Manage complex IT system	Yes	No
Comments:	___no. of years	
• Training program experience	Yes	No
Comments:		
• Written communication skills	Yes	No
Comments:		
• Oral communication skills	Yes	No
Comments:		
Applicant included: ____Cover Letter _____Résumé _____3 References		

Comments:

Recommend Interview   Yes   No

Print Name of Selection Reviewer_____

Signature of Selection Reviewer_____ Date _____

Table 4.7 Common Questions Asked by Interviewees

What is the turnover rate for your company?
How would you characterize your organizational culture?
Do you promote from within the organization?
How do you see me fitting into your organization?
Where do you see your organization in 5 years? 10 years?
What type of training and development do you offer employees?

is used when reviewing a résumé that was submitted to a job posting. The tool uses the posting information as the parameters for determining if an applicant is qualified for a job opening. Using the job posting in Table 4.5 as the basis for the review tool, a panel of reviewers will have standardization when reviewing several applicants.

In addition to the review process, good interviewers should be familiar with potential questions interviewees may ask them about their organization. Table 4.7 provides examples of typical interviewee questions. The HR department can provide training to the interviewers regarding the importance of representing the organization in a professional manner.

■ Hiring Diverse Employees

To attract a diverse pool of applicants, management and HR should develop a recruitment and selection plan. The following are tips that can support the organization as an equal employment opportunity employer:

1. Equal employment opportunity statements: The company should have a diversity policy on its website and on its individual job postings. The statement should easily be found on the website. By including an equal employment opportunity statement on any job posting, regardless of where it is posted, the company makes a statement that it is proactive in creating a diverse work environment. For example, the American College of Healthcare Executives promotes diversity on its website and encourages healthcare organizations to follow its example (Increasing and Sustaining Racial/Ethnic Diversity, 2010).
2. Specialized publications: Placing job postings in magazines and on websites that target specific protected classes will increase the diversity of applicants.
3. Diverse recruiters: Sending diverse recruiters to job fairs that represent different protected classes will encourage diversity in job applicants.
4. Diverse interviewers: During the selection process, continue to demonstrate diversity by selecting a diverse pool of interviewers. This will encourage applicants that are more diverse.

Being proactive in diversity hiring practices will enable the organization to avoid any issues with discrimination. It will also acknowledge the increased diversity of patients in the healthcare industry.

▪ Uniform Guidelines on Employee Selection Procedures

In 1978, the EEOC published the Uniform Guidelines on Employee Selections to ensure there are fair selection processes for all components of selecting employees. The EEOC, the Civil Service Commission, the U.S. Department of Justice, and the U.S. Department of Labor have adopted these guidelines. These guidelines provide information on the issue of unfair selection procedures including disparate treatment and impact. They have been modified over the years to reflect Supreme Court decisions related to employment discrimination (Mondy, 2012).

▪ Disparate Treatment and Disparate Impact

Disparate treatment occurs when protected classes (race, color, religion, sex, or national origin) are treated differently from nonprotected classes. For example, a female candidate who is qualified for a job may be asked to perform a skill or take a test that a male applicant may not take and the male is consequently hired. This applies to all employment procedures including interviews, application forms, **work samples**, physical requirements, and performance evaluations.

Disparate treatment in the selection process occurs through intentional discrimination against a protected group. **Disparate impact** is the underrepresentation of protected classes in an organization's workforce (Fried & Fottler, 2008). Disparate impact is determined by the four-fifths rule: If the selection rate for a protected class is less than four fifths, or less than 80%, of the hiring rate of the majority group, then disparate impact exists (EEOC Selection Guidelines, 2011) (Table 4.8).

▪ Bona Fide Occupational Qualification

There are exceptions to disparate treatment. A **Bona fide occupational qualification** (BFOQ) means that a particular characteristic allows an organization to discriminate against a protected-class individual. Title VII of the Civil Rights Act of 1964 states that employers can discriminate based on gender, religion, or national origin if the characteristic can be considered a BFOQ. Race is not included in this exception. For example, an organization would hire a male attendant for a men's restroom. If a woman applied for the job, she would not be chosen. Religious institutions may decline to hire applicants who have different religious backgrounds than that of the institution (Dessler, 2012). Courts and the EEOC have been hesitant to allow organizations to

Table 4.8 How to Determine if Disparate Impact Exists

Premise: A healthcare organization wants to hire 75 X-ray technicians.

- Of the 200 applicants that apply, 100 are male and 100 are female—all equally qualified.
- The organization hires 50 of the male applicants and 25 of the female applicants.

Step 1: Calculate the hiring rates of each group.

- 50 males hired/100 male applications = 50%, or 0.50
- 25 females hired/100 female applications = 25%, or 0.25

Step 2: Compare the hiring rates.

- The hiring rate of the female applicants was 25%, which means that one out of four female applicants was hired. The hiring rate of the male applicants was 50%, which means that one out of two male applicants was hired.

Step 3: Apply the four-fifths, or 80%, rule.

- Divide the hiring rate of the women (25%) by the hiring rate of the men (50%). The ratio is 50%. If the ratio between the protected class group, which is women in this case, is less than four fifths, or 80%, of the majority group, which is the male group, then disparate impact exists in the hiring process. The result of 50% indicates there is an unfair representation of the protected class (females) in this hiring process, which may indicate a discriminatory process.

prefer one gender to the other. There are exceptions to consumer preferences that are allowed in health care. In the obstetrics/gynecology field, courts have indicated that preferences of consumers are permitted in some instances related to the privacy of their genital areas. The healthcare industry has unique circumstances when it comes to consumer preferences and the comfort of exposing a patient's body. Females may prefer female gynecologists, and, therefore, a healthcare organization may rightfully decline hiring a male gynecologist because of BFOQ (McLaughlin, O'Day & Shorter, 2007). There have not been many cases regarding this issue. It will be interesting to see what happens over the next decade as it relates to health care and consumer privacy.

■ Conclusion

An organization should plan a systematic recruitment process to ensure that appropriate candidates will apply for positions. Organizations can recruit both internally and externally. Regardless of the recruitment method, the organization must assess the effectiveness of the types of chosen recruitment methods. Once the recruitment process has been completed, the next step is to select the appropriate candidates for the organization. Typical selection processes include standardized interviews and, in some instances, employment tests that assess aptitude, attitude, honesty, and personality. These procesess must be legally defensible.

■ Vocabulary

Advertising
Agreeableness
Aptitude tests
Background checks
Behavioral interview
Big Five Personality Traits
Bona fide occupational qualification
Cognitive ability tests
Conscientiousness
Content validity
Correlation coefficient
Criminal background checks
Criterion-validity
Direct methods of recruiting
Disparate impact
Disparate treatment
Educational recruitment
Electronic job recruitment
Emotional stability
External recruitment sources
Extraversion
Healthcare aptitude test
Health on the Net Foundation (HON)

Honesty tests
Identity (attitude and aptitude) tests
Indirect methods of recruiting
Internal recruitment sources
Job postings
Legally defensible
Openness to experience
Personality tests
Physical ability tests
Psychomotor tests
Recruiters
Recruitment
Reliability
Selection process
Shadowing program
Situational interview
Social media
Source yield ratios
Structured interviews
Temporary employment agencies
Unstructured interviews
Validity
Work sample tests

■ References

About Maxim Staffing Solutions. (2011). Available at: http://www.maximstaffing.com/aboutUs/index.aspx. Accessed December 9, 2011.

Arnold, D. (2011). Cognitive ability testing: White paper. Available at: http://www.wonderlic.com. Accessed May 29, 2011.

Byars, L. & Rues, L. (2006). *Human Resource Management* (8th ed.). New York, NY: McGraw-Hill/Irwin, pp. 111, 112, 132–133.

Dessler, G. (2012). *Fundamentals of Human Resource Management.* Upper Saddle River, NJ: Prentice Hall, pp. 100–102.

EEOC Selection Guidelines (2011). Available at: http://www.eeoc.gov/policy/docs/qanda_clarify_procedures.html. Accessed May 29, 2011.

ejobfairs.net (2011). What is an eJobFair? Available at: http://www.ejobfairs.net/index.php?page=whatis. Accessed January 11, 2011.

employtest.com (2011). Healthcare Aptitude Test. Available at: http://www.employtest.com/healthcare-aptitude-test-/. Accessed May 28, 2011.

Fried, B. & Fottler, M. (2008). *Human Resources in Healthcare* (3rd ed.). Chicago, IL: Health Administration Press, pp. 443–449.

Hitt, M., Miller, C. & Colella, A. (2006). *Organizational Behavior: A Strategic Approach.* Hoboken, NJ: Wiley, pp. 160–166.

Homula, M. (2005). *The Great Eight: How to Identify, Select, and Hire Great Recruiters.* Available at: http://www.ere.net/2005/10/11/the-great-eight-how-to-identify-select-and-hire-great-recruiters. Accessed January 11, 2011.

HON Code of Conduct (2011). Available at: http://hon.ch/HONcode/Patients/Conduct.html. Accessed January 10, 2011.

Increasing and Sustaining Racial/Ethnic Diversity in Healthcare Management (2010). Available at: http://www.ache.org/policy/minority.cfm. Accessed May 29, 2011.

Lievens, F., Coetsier, P., Fruyt, F. & De Maesseneer, J. (2002). Medical students' personality characteristics and academic performance: A five-factor model perspective. *Medical Education*, 36:1050–1056.

Mathis, R. & Jackson, J. (2006). *Human Resource Management* (11th ed.). Mason, OH: Thomson/South-Western, pp. 192–223.

McLaughlin, C., O'Day, T. & Shorter, T. (2007). Can we use gender in our hiring decisions? The discrimination bona fide occupational qualification (BFOQ) applied to healthcare. Available at: http://www.gklaw.com/news.cfm?action=pub_details&publication_id=544. Accessed January 17, 2011.

Mondy, R. (2012). *Human Resource Managemeent* (12th ed.). Upper Saddle River, NJ: Prentice Hall, pp. 66–70.

Noe, R., Hollenbeck, J., Gerhart, B. & Wright, P. (2012a). *Fundamentals of Human Resource Management* (3rd ed). New York, NY: McGraw-Hill/Irwin, pp. 136–137.

Noe, R., Hollenbeck, J., Gerhart, B. & Wright, P., (2012b). *Fundamentals of Human Resource Management* (3rd ed). New York, NY: McGraw-Hill/Irwin, pp. 163–167.

Shermont, H. & Murphy, J. (2006). Shadowing: A winning recruitment tool. *Nursing Management*, November. Available at: http://www.nursing management.com. Accessed November 1, 2010.

Source Yield (2011). Available at: http://www.shrm.org/Research/Articles/Articles/Pages/MetricoftheMonthSourceYield.aspx. Accessed December 10, 2011.

totaltesting.com (2011). Attitude and Aptitude (Identity) Tests. Available at: http://www.totaltesting.com/aptitude-attitude-tests.shtml. Accessed May 29, 2011.

STUDENT WORKBOOK ACTIVITY 4.1

Complete the following case scenarios based on the information provided in the chapter. Your answers must be *in your own words*.

Real-Life Applications: Case Scenario 1

You have been asked by your supervisor to develop a plan to recruit for 10 nursing positions for your hospital. She wants you to use both internal and external recruiting sources.

Activity

Discuss the different types of recruitment sources you will be using for this plan. Be specific. Identify an advantage and disadvantage of internal and external recruiting sources.

Responses

_____

_____

_____

_____

_____

Real-Life Applications: Case Scenario 2

You have been asked to work with the HR department to develop a training program for recruiters.

Activity

Review the concept of source yield ratio to ensure the recruiting plans are effective. Include a specific example of how to calculate this ratio, and the ratio of disparate treatment.

Responses

_____

_____

_____

_____

Real-Life Applications: Case Scenario 3

Your supervisor asks you to be an interviewer for a medical illustrator position that is now vacant.

Activity

Review the responsibilities of the position. Develop a recruitment and selection plan to fill the position.

Responses

_____

_____

_____

_____

Real-Life Applications: Case Scenario 4

The CEO would like to increase the organization's ethical commitment. He has heard that the Cleveland Clinic is certified by some health organization for ethical behavior.

Activity

Research the Health on the Net Foundation and provide your CEO with information regarding its goals and activities that would fit with your organization.

Responses

_____

_____

_____

_____

_____

STUDENT WORKBOOK ACTIVITY 4.2

In Your Own Words

Please describe these core concepts in your own words.

Disparate treatment:

_____

_____

_____

_____

Disparate impact:

_____

_____

_____

_____

Validity:

_____

_____

_____

_____

Reliability:

_____

_____

_____

_____

Bona fide occupational qualification:

_____

_____

_____

_____

Source yield ratio:

_____

_____

_____

_____

Big Five Personality Traits:

_____

_____

_____

_____

Social media:

_____

_____

_____

_____

Correlation coefficient:

_____

_____

_____

_____

STUDENT WORKBOOK ACTIVITY 4.3

Internet Exercises

Write your answers in the spaces provided.

- Visit each of the websites listed in the text that follows.
- Name the organization.
- Locate its mission statement on its website. If the organization does not have a mission statement, describe its purpose.
- Provide a brief overview of the activities of the organization.
- Apply this organization to the chapter information.

Websites

http://www.ache.org

Organization name:

_____

Mission statement:

_____

_____

_____

Overview of activities:

_____

_____

_____

Application to chapter information:

_____

_____

_____

http://www.healthlinesystems.com

Organization name:

_____

Mission statement:

_____

_____

_____

Overview of activities:

_____

_____

_____

Application to chapter information:

_____

_____

_____

http://careeronestop.com

Organization name:

_____

Mission statement:

_____

_____

_____

Overview of activities:

_____

_____

_____

Application to chapter information:

_____

_____

_____

http://www.nursingmanagement.com
Organization name:

_____

Mission statement:

_____

_____

_____

Overview of activities:

_____

_____

_____

Application to chapter information:

_____

_____

_____

http://www.hon.ch
Organization name:

_____

Mission statement:

_____

_____

_____

Overview of activities:

_____

_____

_____

Application to chapter information:

_____

_____

_____

http://www.eeoc.gov

Organization name:

_____

Mission statement:

_____

_____

_____

Overview of activities:

_____

_____

_____

Application to chapter information:

_____

_____

_____

STUDENT ACTIVITY 4.4: DISCUSSION BOARDS FOR ONLINE, HYBRID, AND TRADITIONAL CLASSES

Discussion Board Guidelines

The discussion board is used in online and web-enhanced courses in place of classroom lectures and discussion. The board can also be used as an enhancement to traditional classes. The discussion board is the way in which the students "link together" as a class. The following are guidelines to help focus on the discussion topic and to define the roles and responsibilities of the discussion coordinator and other members of the class. The educator will be the discussion moderator for this course.

1. The educator will post the discussion topic and directions for the upcoming week. These postings should all be responses to the original topic or responses to other students' responses. When people respond to what someone else has posted, they should start the posting with the person's name so it is clear which message they are responding to. **A response such as "Yes" or "I agree" does not count for credit. Your responses must be in your own words. You cannot copy and paste from the text.**
2. Postings (especially responses) should include enough information so the message is clear but should not be so long that it becomes difficult to follow. Remember, this is like talking to someone in a classroom setting. The postings should reflect the content of the text or other assignments. If you retrieve information from the Internet, the hyperlink must be cited.
3. Students should check the discussion daily to see if new information has been posted that requires their attention and response.

Good discussion will often include different points of view. Students should feel free to disagree or "challenge" others to support their positions or ideas. All discussions must be handled in a respectful manner. The following are discussion boards for this chapter.

Discussion Boards

1. What is recruitment? Which is more important, internal or external? Or are both equally important? Defend your answer.
2. What do you think of social media as a recruitment tool?
3. What is shadowing? Do you think this is a valuable way to recruit in the health-care industry? Would you participate in this process? Defend your answer.
4. Discuss different selection tests. Have you ever taken a selection test? Do you think these tests are a good way to select employees? Defend your answer.

Training and Developing the Organization

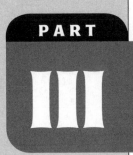

Careers in Health Care

The student will be able to:

- Identify five types of physicians and their roles in health care.
- Discuss six types of nurse professionals and their roles in health care.
- Evaluate six types of other health professionals and their roles in health care.
- Examine the role of allied health professionals in the healthcare industry.
- Assess five certified allied health education programs.

DID YOU KNOW THAT?

- The healthcare industry is one of the largest employers in the United States.
- Approximately 59% of U.S. physicians are specialists (surgeons, cardiologists, etc.).
- Medicare is the principal source of funding for graduate medical education.
- Since the 1990s, physicians who specialize in the care of hospitalized patients have been referred to as "hospitalists."
- Nurses are the largest group of healthcare professionals in the United States.

■ Introduction

The healthcare industry is one of the largest employers in the United States and employs more than 3% of the U.S. workforce. There are approximately 200 health occupations and professions in a workforce of more than 12 million healthcare workers. By 2030, the percentage of the population that is 65 years and older will increase from the current 6% to 10% of the total population, which will place pressure on the healthcare system (National Center for Health Statistics, 2008). Because of the aging of our population, the Bureau of Labor Statistics (BLS) indicates that health care will generate more than 3 million new jobs by 2018 (BLS, 2011a). When one thinks of healthcare providers, one automatically thinks of physicians and nurses. However, the healthcare industry is composed of many different health services professionals, such as dentists, optometrists, psychologists, chiropractors, podiatrists, non-physician practitioners (NPPs), administrators, and allied health professionals. Allied health professionals, who represent 60% of the healthcare workforce, provide a range of essential healthcare services that complement the services provided by physicians and nurses (Shi & Singh, 2008).

Health care can occur in varied settings. Many physicians have their own practices, but they may also work in hospitals, mental health facilities, managed care organizations, or community health centers. They may also hold government positions, teach at a university, or be employed by an insurance company. Health professionals, in general, may work at many different for-profit and not-for-profit organizations. However, hospitals employ 35% of all healthcare employees (BLS, 2011b). In most states, only physicians, dentists, and a few other practitioners may serve patients directly without the authorization of another licensed independent health professional. Those categories authorized include chiropractic, optometry, psychotherapy, and podiatry. There also continues to be a shortage of nurses nationwide. It is projected that nursing shortages will continue to lag 36% behind nursing staffing needs (Bradley, 2008). It is the responsibility of the human resources (HR) department to be aware of the different types of healthcare jobs in the industry. When employees transfer within an organization or decide to change their healthcare career goals, their main resource is the HR department. This chapter will provide a description of the different types of healthcare jobs, their educational requirements, job responsibilities and average salaries, and their roles in the healthcare system.

■ Physician Education

Physicians play a major role in providing healthcare services. Physicians diagnose and treat patient illnesses. All states require a license to practice medicine. Physicians must receive their medical education from an accredited school that awards either a **doctor of medicine** (MD) or a **doctor of osteopathic medicine** (DO) degree. Many students prepare for medical school by majoring in a premedical undergraduate program, which often consists of science and mathematics. Undergraduate students are also required to take the Medical College Admission Test (MCAT). In 2008, there existed 129 accredited U.S. medical schools that awarded the doctor of medicine degree (BLS, 2011c). To provide direct patient care, the physician must take a licensing examination in the desired state of practice once he or she completes a residency. State licensing requirements may vary. The residency is important because it allows physicians to learn about a certain specialty of interest while providing them with on-the-job training. The length of the residency program can be as short as 3 years for a family practice and as long as 10 years for different surgery specialties. There exist residency programs that are hospital based, community based, and university affiliated. The American Medical Association has an online database of all accredited residency programs by state and location. Most states require physicians to participate in continuing medical education activities to maintain state licensure (Sultz & Young, 2006; Buchbinder & Shanks, 2007; Pointer et al., 2008; Shi & Singh, 2008).

In 2008, there existed only 25 accredited medical schools that conferred the DO degree (BLS, 2011d). Their enrollment, however, has doubled over the past 20 years. DOs represent approximately 5% of all U.S. physicians (Sultz & Young, 2006). The major difference between an MD and a DO is in their approaches to treatment. DOs tend to stress preventive treatments and use a holistic approach to treatment, which means they do not focus only on the disease but on the entire person. Most DOs are generalists. MDs use an **allopathic approach,** which means MDs actively intervene in attacking and eradicating disease and focus their efforts on the disease. Most MDs are considered specialists (Pointer et al., 2008; Shi & Singh, 2008).

■ Generalists and Specialists

Generalists are also called primary care physicians. Family care practitioners are also called generalists, as are general internal medicine physicians and general pediatricians. Their focus is preventive services such as immunizations and health examinations. They treat less severe medical problems. They often serve as a gatekeeper for a patient, which means they coordinate patient care if the patient needs to see a specialist for more complex medical problems. **Specialists** are physicians who receive a certification in their area of specialization. This may require additional years of training, as discussed earlier, and **board certification,** or a **credentialing examination.** The most common specialties are dermatology, cardiology, pediatrics, pathology, psychiatry, obstetrics, anesthesiology, specialized internal medicine, gynecology, ophthalmology, radiology, and surgery (Shi & Singh, 2008). The board certification is often associated with the quality of the healthcare provider's services because board certification requires more training. A consumer may view a physician's credentials in the **National Practitioner Data Bank.** This database was created to provide a nationwide system to prohibit incompetent healthcare practitioners from moving state-to-state without disclosure of any previous adverse issues (Buchbinder & Shanks, 2007).

■ Types of Healthcare Providers

Hospitalists

A **hospitalist** is a physician that provides care to hospitalized patients. The hospitalist replaces a patient's primary care physician while the patient is hospitalized.

A hospitalist monitors the patient from admittance to discharge and usually does not have a professional relationship with the patient prior to admittance. This new type of physician, which evolved in the 1990s, is usually a general practitioner and is becoming more popular: Because the hospitalist spends so much time in the hospital setting, he or she can provide care that is more efficient. From a hospital's viewpoint, the focus is maximization of profit, which means shorter lengths of stay, decreased complications, and increased patient satisfaction (Sultz & Young, 2006). There are approximately 12,000 hospitalists in the United States, a number that is expected to triple by 2015. Although they are not board certified as a specialty, they have their own medical journal, annual meetings, and association. This concept has proved to be very effective (Shi & Singh, 2008).

Non-physician Practitioners

Non-physician practitioners (NPPs), which include non-physician clinicians and mid-level practitioners, are sometimes called **physician extenders** because they often are used as substitutes for physicians. They are not involved in total care of a patient, but they collaborate closely with physicians. Categories of NPPs include physician assistants, nurse practitioners, and certified nurse practitioners (Shi & Singh, 2008). NPPs have been favorably received by patients because they tend to spend more time with patients. They play an important role in areas that have physician shortages such as certain urban areas, community health centers, and the managed care environment. NPPs can perform repetitive technical tasks such as disease screenings. They may also take care of non–life-threatening cases in emergency departments and perform physicals, drug testing, and other routine activities. Their salaries are nearly 50% less than physician salaries, so they are a cost-effective patient caregiver. As NPPs become more involved in patient care, reimbursement for their services should be addressed. At this time, reimbursement is usually directed toward their collaborating physician, which often results in payment delays. As the roles of NPPs increase in patient care because of cost-cutting measures by healthcare organizations, regulations and guidelines must be updated and maintained to ensure high-quality patient care by NPPs (Shi & Singh, 2008).

Physician Assistants

Physician assistants (PAs), a category of NPP, provide a range of diagnostic and therapeutic services to patients. They take medical histories, conduct patient examinations, analyze tests, make diagnoses, and perform basic medical procedures. They are able to prescribe medicines in all but three states. They must be associated with and supervised by a physician, but the supervision does not need to be direct. In areas where there is a physician shortage, PAs act as primary care providers. They collaborate with physicians by telephone and on-site visits. There are 129 accredited 2-year PA programs in the United States. Many students have previous healthcare experience. They are required to pass a national certification exam. They may take additional education in surgery, pediatrics, emergency medicine, primary care, and occupational medicine. The average yearly PA salary is $65,000. Their employment growth is expected to be 40% by 2018 (BLS, 2011e).

■ Types of Nurses

Registered nurses constitute the largest group of healthcare professionals. Nurses provide the majority of care to patients, accounting for 26% of the U.S. workforce (BLS, 2011f). They are the patient's advocate. There are several different types of nurses that provide patient care, and there are several different levels of nursing care based on education and training. The following sections summarize the various types of nurses.

Licensed Practical Nurses or Licensed Vocational Nurses (California and Texas)

There are approximately 700,000 **licensed practical nurses** (LPNs) in the United States, and they represent the largest group of nurses. Education for LPNs is offered by community colleges or technical schools. Training takes approximately 12–14 months and includes both education and supervised clinical practice. There are 1,100 LPN programs in the United States. LPNs have a high school diploma and take a licensing exam. The yearly LPN salary is approximately $29,000. Their job responsibilities include observing patients, taking vital signs, keeping records, assisting patients with personal hygiene, and feeding and dressing patients, which are considered **activities of daily living** (ADLs). In some states, LPNs administer some medications. They work primarily in hospitals, home health agencies, and nursing homes. Many LPNs work full-time and earn their bachelor of science in nursing (BSN) to increase their career choices (BLS, 2011b).

Registered Nurses

There are approximately 2.5 million registered nurses (RNs) in the United States, and they represent the largest healthcare occupation, with greater than 55% working in hospitals. An RN is a graduate trained nurse who has been licensed by a state board after passing the national nursing examination. RNs can be registered in more than one state, and there are different levels of RN based on education.

The **associate degree in nursing** (ADN) is a 2-year program offered by community colleges and some 4-year universities. Many students obtain an ADN and continue their education to receive a BSN degree. There are also 3-year diploma programs for ADNs, which are offered by hospitals. The programs are expensive and are being offered less often. There are approximately 70 diploma programs left in the United States.

The **bachelor of science in nursing** (BSN) is the most rigorous of the nursing programs. These programs offered by colleges and universities usually take 4–5 years to complete, and the students perform both classroom activity and clinical practice activity. Their job responsibilities include recording symptoms of any disease, implementing care plans, assisting physicians in examination and treatment of patients, administering medications and performing medical procedures, supervising other personnel such as LPNs, and educating patients and families about follow-up care. The majority of RNs work in hospitals, and the average annual income for these individuals is $62,000 but varies depending on the level of education.

The **advanced practical nurse** (APN), or midlevel practitioner, is a nurse who has experience and education beyond the requirements of an RN. The responsibilities of an APN exist between those of the RN and MD, which is why they are called **midlevel practitioners**. APNs typically obtain a master of science in nursing with a specialty in the field of practice. There are four areas of specialization: clinical nurse specialist, certified registered nurse anesthetist, nurse practitioner, and certified nurse midwife. Many of these certifications allow a nurse to provide direct care including writing of prescriptions (BLS, 2011e).

Nurse Practitioners and Certified Nurse Midwives

As stated earlier, NPPs are integral to the provision of quality health care in the United States. **Nurse practitioners** (NPs) represent the largest category of APNs. The first group of NPs was trained in 1965 at the University of Colorado. In 1974, the American Nursing Association developed the Council of Primary Care Nurse Practitioners, which helped substantiate the role of NPs in patient care. Over the past two decades, several specialty NP boards have been established, such as pediatrics and reproductive health, for certification of NPs. In 1985, the American Association of Nurse Practitioners was established as a professional organization for NPs. The median salary of a nurse practitioner is $89,899. As of 2007, there were approximately 120,000 practicing NPs with an average of 6,000 NPs receiving training at more than 325 educational institutions (American Academy of Nurse Practitioners, 2008). They are required to obtain an RN and a master's degree. They may participate in a certificate program and complete direct patient care clinical training. NPs emphasize health education and promotion as well as disease treatment—referred to as care and cure. They spend more time with patients, and, as a result, patient surveys indicate satisfaction with care from NPs. They may specialize in pediatric, family, geriatric, or psychiatric care. Most states allow NPs to prescribe medications. Recent statistics indicate that 600 million visits are made to NPs annually (American Academy of Nurse Practitioners, 2008).

Certified nurse midwives (CNMs) are RNs who have graduated from a nurse midwifery education program that has been accredited by the American College of Nurse-Midwives' Division of Accreditation. Nurse midwives are primary care providers for women who are pregnant. Nurse midwives have been practicing in the United States for nearly 90 years. They must pass the national certification exam to receive the designation of CNM, and they must be recertified every 8 years. The average annual salary is $91,535. **Certified midwives** (CMs) are individuals who do not have a nursing degree but have a related health background. They must take the midwifery education program, which is accredited by the same organization. They must also pass the same national certification exam to be given the designation of CM. The average annual salary for a CM is $61,000 (BLS, 2011e).

Certified Nursing Assistants or Aides

Certified nursing assistants (CNAs) are unlicensed patient attendants who work under the supervision of physicians and nurses. They answer patient call bells and assist patients in personal hygiene, bed change, meal orders, and ADLs. Most CNAs are employed by nursing care facilities. There are approximately 1.5 million CNAs in the healthcare industry. They are required to receive 75 hours of training and are required to pass a competency examination. Their average pay is extremely low. The annual median salary is $28,368. They are often overlooked for advancement, and therefore there is a high turnover in their field (Pointer, Williams, Isaacs & Knickman, 2007; Shi & Singh, 2008).

■ Nursing Shortages

Although nursing supply and demand is cyclical, during recent years there has continued to be a nursing shortage. The current shortage began a decade ago, making it the longest shortage in 50 years. According to the BLS, employment of RNs will increase by 22% by 2016. Without recruitment for nursing programs, the Health and Human Services Administration projects the supply of U.S. nurses will lag 36% behind nursing staffing needs (Bradley, 2008). Although community colleges have developed quality nursing programs nationally, there is increased pressure for students to obtain additional nursing education. One reason why there is a shortage of nursing personnel is the lack of qualified nursing faculty available. Unlike faculty members in other disciplines who generally have doctorates, approximately 50% of faculty members in BSN and advanced degree programs do not hold a doctorate. Many nursing faculty members leave for wage increases in the clinical and private sectors. The average yearly salary for a member of a nursing faculty is $62,000. NPs who own their own practices earn an average of $94,000 per year (Yordy, 2006).

■ Other Independent Healthcare Professionals

Dentists

Dentists prevent, diagnose, and treat tooth, gum, and mouth diseases. They are required to complete 4 years of education at an accredited dental school after a bachelor's degree has been completed. In 2008, there were 57 accredited dental schools. Dentists are awarded a doctor of dental surgery or doctor of dental medicine degree. Some states may require a specialty license. The first 2 years of dental school are focused on dental sciences, and the last 2 years are spent in a clinical environment. Dentists may take an additional 2–4 years of postgraduate education in eight different specialties. There are nearly 140,000 dentists in the United States—more than 90% are in private practice and are primarily general practitioners. The average annual income for dentists is $143,000 (BLS, 2011f). Dental practices are not part of a managed care environment. Dentists only serve those who have dental insurance or who can pay out of pocket. There are sections of underserved populations that will continue to be underserved because there is no industry priority to target those populations (Sultz & Young, 2006).

Dentists are often helped by **dental hygienists** and **dental assistants**. Dental hygienists clean teeth and educate patients on proper dental care. In order to practice, dental hygienists must be licensed, which requires graduation from an accredited dental hygienist school and passing of both national and state licensing exams. Dental assistants work directly with dentists in the preparation and treatment of patients. They do not have to be licensed, but there are certification programs available (BLS, 2011a).

Pharmacists

Pharmacists are responsible for dispensing prescribed medication. They also advise both patients and healthcare providers about potential side effects of medications. Pharmacists must earn a PharmD degree from an accredited college or school of pharmacy, which has replaced the bachelor of pharmacy degree. To be admitted to a PharmD program, an applicant must complete at least 2 years of postsecondary study, although most applicants have completed 3 or more years, which include courses in mathematics and natural sciences. In 2007, 92 colleges and schools of pharmacy were accredited to confer degrees. There are approximately 70 U.S. pharmacy schools that confer the PharmD degree. The students who complete the PharmD degree may opt to complete 1- to 2-year residencies or fellowships that are designed for those who want specialized pharmaceutical training. Pharmacists who want to work in a clinical setting are often required to complete a residency.

In 2008, there were nearly 270,000 active U.S. pharmacists—approximately 60% of them working in community pharmacies. Approximately 25% of pharmacists work in hospitals, with the remaining 15% working in physicians' offices, mail order and Internet pharmacies, nursing homes, and the federal government. In 2008, the mean annual salary for a pharmacist was $106,000 (BLS, 2011g).

Chiropractors

Chiropractors have a holistic approach to treating their patients. They believe that the body can heal itself without medication or surgery. Their focus is the entire body, emphasizing the spine. They manipulate the body with their hands or with a machine. Chiropractors must be licensed, which requires 2–4 years of undergraduate education, the completion of a 4-year chiropractic college course, and passing scores on national and state examinations. In 2009, 16 chiropractic programs and 2 chiropractic institutions in the United States were accredited by the Council on Chiropractic Education. Applicants must have at least 90 semester hours of undergraduate study leading toward a bachelor's degree before entering the program. Chiropractic programs require a minimum of 4,200 hours of classroom, laboratory, and clinical experience. During the first 2 years, most chiropractic programs emphasize classroom learning and laboratory experience. The last 2 years focus on courses in manipulation and spinal adjustment and clinical experience. Chiropractic programs and institutions grant the doctor of chiropractic degree. In 2009, there were 49,000 chiropractors in the United States. In 2009, the mean salary for a chiropractor was $94,000 (BLS, 2011h).

Optometrists

Optometrists, also known as doctors of optometry, are the main providers of vision care. They examine people's eyes to diagnose vision problems. Optometrists may prescribe eyeglasses or contact lenses. Optometrists also test for glaucoma and other eye diseases and diagnose conditions caused by systemic diseases, such as diabetes and high blood pressure, and refer patients to other health practitioners. Optometrists often provide preoperative and postoperative care to cataract patients and to patients who have had laser vision correction or other eye surgery.

Optometrists must obtain a doctor of optometry degree, which requires the completion of a 4-year program at an accredited optometry school. In 2009, there were 19 colleges of optometry in the United States and 1 in Puerto Rico that offered accredited programs. Requirements for admission to optometry schools include college courses in English, mathematics, physics, chemistry, and biology. Because a strong background in science is important, many applicants to optometry school major in a science as undergraduates. Admission to optometry school is competitive. Applicants must take the Optometry Admissions Test, which measures academic ability and scientific comprehension. As a result, most applicants take the test after their sophomore or junior year in college, allowing them an opportunity to take the test again and raise their scores. However, most students accepted by a school or college of optometry have completed an undergraduate degree (BLS, 2011i).

All states require that optometrists be licensed. Applicants for a license must have a doctor of optometry degree from an accredited optometry school and must pass both a written national board examination and a national, regional, or state clinical examination. Many states also require applicants to pass an examination on relevant state laws. Licenses must be renewed every 1–3 years, and, in all states, continuing education credits are needed for renewal. Optometrists held about 35,000 jobs in 2008. Employment of optometrists is expected to grow in response to the vision care needs of a growing and aging population. The median annual salary for optometrists was $96,000 in 2008 (BLS, 2011i).

Psychologists

Psychologists study the human mind and human behavior. Research psychologists investigate the physical, cognitive, emotional, or social aspects of human behavior. Psychologists in health service fields provide mental health care in hospitals, clinics, schools, or private settings. Psychologists are employed in applied settings such as business, industry, government, or nonprofit organizations and provide training, conduct research, design organizational systems, and act as advocates for psychology. They usually specialize in one of a number of different areas.

Clinical psychologists—who represent the largest specialty—work most often in counseling centers, independent or group practices, hospitals, or clinics. They help mentally and emotionally distressed clients and may assist medical patients in dealing with illnesses or injuries. Areas of specialization within clinical psychology include health psychology, neuropsychology, and geropsychology. Health psychologists study how biological, psychological, and social factors affect health and illness. Neuropsychologists study the relation between the brain and behavior. They often work in stroke and head injury programs. Geropsychologists deal with the special problems faced by the elderly. Often, clinical psychologists consult with other medical personnel regarding the best treatment for patients, especially treatment that includes medication. Unlike psychiatrists and other medical doctors, clinical psychologists generally are not permitted to prescribe medication. However, Louisiana and New Mexico currently allow certain clinical psychologists to prescribe medication with some limitations.

Counseling psychologists use various techniques, including interviewing and testing, to advise people on how to deal with career or work problems and problems faced in different stages of life. School psychologists work with students in early childhood and elementary and secondary schools. School psychologists address students' learning and behavioral problems, suggest improvements to classroom management strategies or parenting techniques, and evaluate students with disabilities and gifted and talented students to help determine the best way to educate them.

Industrial-organizational psychologists apply psychological principles and research methods to the workplace in the interest of improving productivity and the quality of work life. Developmental psychologists study the physiologic, cognitive, and social development that takes place throughout life. Some specialize in behavior during infancy, childhood, and adolescence or changes that occur during maturity or old age. **Social psychologists** examine people's interactions with others and with the social environment. **Experimental** or **research psychologists** work in university and private research centers and in business, nonprofit, and government organizations.

A doctoral degree usually is required for independent practice as a psychologist. Psychologists with a PhD or doctor of psychology (PsyD) degree qualify for a wide range of teaching, research, clinical, and counseling positions in universities, healthcare services, elementary and secondary schools, private industry, and government. Psychologists with these doctoral degrees (PhD or PsyD) often work in clinical positions or in private practices, but they may teach, conduct research, or become administrators. These doctoral degrees generally require 5–7 years of graduate study, culminating in a dissertation based on original research. The PsyD degree may be based on practical work and examinations rather than a dissertation. In clinical, counseling, and school psychology, the requirements for these degrees include at least a 1-year internship. Psychologists held approximately 170,000 jobs in 2008. Educational institutions employed about 30% of psychologists in positions such as counseling, testing, research, and administration. About 21% were employed in health care, primarily in offices of mental health. Government agencies at the state and local levels employed psychologists primarily in correctional facilities and law enforcement (BLS, 2011j).

Podiatrists

Podiatrists treat patients for foot diseases and deformities. They are awarded a doctor of podiatric medicine (PDM) degree upon completion of a 4-year podiatric graduate program. At least 90 hours of undergraduate education and acceptable scores on the MCAT, Dental Admission Test, or the Graduate Record Exam are needed to enter a PDM degree program. In 2008, there were eight colleges of podiatric medicine accredited by the Council on Podiatric Medical Education. Their curriculum is similar to that of other schools of medicine. Most graduates complete a residency in a hospital, which lasts 2–4 years. All states require a license to practice podiatric medicine. Podiatrists may also be board certified in their chosen specialties. All podiatrists must pass a national examination by their national board. Established in 1912, the American Podiatric Medical Association is the premier professional organization representing the nation's doctors of podiatric medicine (BLS, 2011).

Generally, podiatrists may perform surgeries, prescribe medications and corrective devices such as orthoses, and provide therapies. Many chronic diseases such as arthritis and diabetes exhibit symptoms in the feet of patient, so podiatrists may coordinate their efforts with other healthcare providers. Podiatrists' specializations include areas of sports medicine, geriatrics, or diabetes, and they may be board certified in their specialty, which requires advanced training. Most podiatrists work in private practice and treat fewer emergencies than other doctors. Some podiatrists serve on the staffs of hospitals and long-term care facilities, teach in schools of medicine, serve as commissioned officers in the Armed Forces and the U.S. Public Health Service and the Department of Veterans Affairs, and work in state health departments (American

Podiatric Medical Association, 2008). Many operate in solo practices, but recent trends indicate they are forming group practices. According to 2008 BLS statistics, there are more than 12,000 podiatrists nationwide with a 2008 median annual salary of $113,000 (BLS, 2011).

■ Allied Health Professionals

In the early 20th century, healthcare providers consisted of physicians, nurses, pharmacists, and optometrists. As the healthcare industry evolved with increased use of technology and sophisticated interventions, increased time demands were placed on these healthcare providers. As a result, a broader spectrum of healthcare professionals evolved with skills that complemented those of the primary healthcare providers. These **allied health professionals** assist physicians and nurses in providing care to their patients. They provide both direct and indirect patient care. There are 5 million allied health professionals in the United States who work in 80 different professions and represent nearly 60% of the healthcare workforce (Allied Health Professions Overview, 2012). The impact of technology has increased the number of different specialties available. They can be divided into four main categories: laboratory technologists and technicians, therapeutic science practitioners, behavioral scientists, and support services (Association of Schools of Allied Health Professionals, 2009).

Laboratory technologists and technicians have a major role in diagnosing disease, assessing the impact of interventions, and applying highly technical procedures. Examples of this category include radiologic technology and nuclear medicine technology. Therapeutic science practitioners focus on the rehabilitation of patients with diseases and injuries. Examples of this category include physical therapists, radiation therapists, respiratory therapists, dieticians, and dental hygienists. Behavioral scientists such as social workers and rehabilitation counselors provide social, psychological, and community and patient educational activities (Sultz & Young, 2006). This chapter cannot describe all allied health professional and support services programs, but a list of accredited allied health careers will be discussed.

The Commission on Accreditation of Allied Health Education Programs (CAAHEP) accredits 2,000 U.S. education programs that offer more than 20 allied health specialties. This section will provide a brief summary of the different accredited allied health education programs that contribute to the provision of quality health care. This information was obtained from the CAAHEP website (CAAHEP, 2011a).

Anesthesiologist Assistant

Under the direction of an anesthesiologist, the **anesthesiologist assistant** is a member of the anesthesia care team for surgical procedures. This specialty physician assistant assists with implementing an anesthesia care plan. Activities include performing presurgical and surgical tasks and possibly also administrative and educational activities. The anesthesiologist assistant primarily is employed by medical centers. As of 2006, starting salaries ranged from $95,000 to $120,000 for 40 hours per week. Acceptance into an anesthesiologist assistant education program requires an undergraduate premedical education. The length of duration of the program is 24–27 months (CAAHEP, 2011b).

Cardiovascular Technologist

At the request of a physician, the **cardiovascular technologist** performs diagnostic examinations for cardiovascular issues. They assist physicians in treating cardiac (heart) and peripheral vascular (blood vessels) problems. They also review and/or record clinical data, perform procedures, and obtain data for physician review. They provide services in any medical setting but primarily are in hospitals. They also operate and maintain testing equipment and may explain test procedures. In 2010, their annual wages ranged from $36,000 to $45,000. Employment of cardiovascular technologists and technicians is expected to increase by 26% through the year 2016. A high school diploma or qualification in a clinically related allied position is required to enter a cardiovascular technologist education program, which may last from 1 to 4 years depending on the background of the student (CAAHEP, 2011c).

Cytotechnologist

Cytology is the study of how cells function and their structure. **Cytotechnologists**, a category of clinical laboratory technologists, are specialists who collaborate with pathologists to evaluate cellular material. This material is used by pathologists to diagnose diseases, such as cancer. Most cytotechnologists work in hospitals. Employment of clinical laboratory workers such as cytotechnologists is expected to grow by 14% by 2016. In 2007, wages for clinical laboratory technologists averaged $30 per hour. To enter a clinical laboratory technologist education program, applicants should have a background in the biological sciences. Applicants must have an undergraduate degree to qualify for national certification (CAAHEP, 2011d).

Diagnostic Medical Sonographer

Under the supervision of a physician, a **diagnostic medical sonographer** provides patient services using medical ultrasound, which photographs internal structures. **Sonography** uses sound waves to generate images of the body for the assessment and diagnosis of various medical conditions. Sonography commonly is associated with obstetrics and the use of ultrasound imaging during pregnancy. This specialist gathers data to assist with disease management in a variety of medical facilities including hospitals, clinics, and private practices. A diagnostic medical sonographer may assist with patient education. In addition to working directly with patients, diagnostic medical sonographers keep patient records.

Diagnostic medical sonographers may specialize in obstetric and gynecologic sonography (the female reproductive system), abdominal sonography (the liver, kidneys, gallbladder, spleen, and pancreas), neurosonography (the brain), breast sonography, vascular sonography, or cardiac sonography. Employment of diagnostic medical sonographers is expected to increase by about 19% through 2016. In 2008, their salaries averaged $43,000. Colleges and universities offer formal training in both 2- and 4-year programs, culminating in an associate's or a bachelor's degree. Applicants to a 1-year education program must have relevant clinical experience. There exist 2-year programs, which are the most prevalent, that will accept high school graduates with an education in basic sciences (CAAHEP, 2011e).

Electroneurodiagnostic Technologist

The **electroneurodiagnostic technologist** is involved with the activity of the brain and nervous system. Electroneurodiagnostic technologists work with physicians and other health professionals. The technologist may take medical histories, document the clinical conditions of patients, and be involved in the diagnostic procedures of the patients. They work primarily in neurology departments of hospitals but may also work in private practices of neurosurgeons and neurologists. In 2006, their annual salary averaged $35,000. Electroneurodiagnostic technologist education programs vary from 12 to 24 months and are offered at community colleges as part of an associate's degree. Applicants must have a high school diploma or equivalent to enter the program (CAAHEP, 2011f).

Emergency Medical Technician–Paramedic

People who are ill, have had an accident, or have been wounded often depend on the competent care of **emergency medical technicians** (EMTs) and paramedics. These patients all require immediate medical attention. EMTs and paramedics provide this vital service as they care for and transport the sick or injured to a medical facility for appropriate medical care. In general, EMTs and EMT–paramedics provide emergency medical assistance that is needed because of an accident or illness that has occurred outside the medical setting. EMTs and paramedics work under guidelines approved by the physician medical director of their healthcare organization to assess and manage medical emergencies. They are trained to provide life-saving measures. EMTs provide basic life support, and EMT–paramedics provide advanced life support measures. They may be employed by an ambulance company, fire department, public emergency medical service (EMS) company, hospital, or a combination thereof. They may be paid or be volunteers from the community. Both EMTs and EMT–paramedics must be proficient in cardiopulmonary resuscitation (CPR). They learn the basics of different types of medical emergencies. EMT–paramedics perform procedures that are more sophisticated. They also receive extensive training in patient assessment. The work is not only physically demanding but also can be stressful, sometimes involving life-or-death situations. In 2006, their average annual salary was approximately $27,000. Firefighters may also be trained as EMTs. EMT training is offered at community colleges, technical schools, hospitals, and academies. EMT training requires 40 hours of training. EMT–paramedics require 200–400 hours of training. Applicants for the programs are expected to have a high school diploma or the equivalent. The National Registry of Emergency Medical Technicians certifies emergency medical service providers at five levels: First Responder, EMT-Basic, EMT-Intermediate (which has two levels called 1985 and 1999), and Paramedic. All 50 states require certification for each of the EMT levels (CAAHEP, 2011g).

Exercise Physiologist

Exercise physiologists assess, design, and manage individual exercise programs for both healthy and unhealthy individuals. Clinical exercise physiologists work with a physician when applying to patients exercise programs that have demonstrated a therapeutic benefit. In 2006, their average wages, depending on geographic area and experience, ranged from $17 to $23 per hour. These allied health professionals may work with fitness trainers, exercise science professionals, or physicians involved with cardiac rehabilitation in hospital settings. Applicants for the 2-year education program should have an undergraduate degree in exercise science (CAAHEP, 2011h).

Exercise Scientist

Exercise scientists focus on biomechanics, nutrition, sports psychology, and exercise physiology. Exercise scientists work in the fitness and health industry. They perform risk assessments, assess health behaviors, and motivate individuals to change negative behaviors. Their program can be completed in a 4-year undergraduate degree. Applicants must have a high school diploma or equivalent (CAAHEP, 2011i).

Kinesiotherapist

Kinesiotherapy is the application of exercise science to enhance the physical capabilities of individuals with limited functions. The **kinesiotherapist** provides rehabilitation exercises as prescribed by a physician. Kinesiotherapists design programs that will reverse, stabilize, or enhance the physical capabilities of patients. They establish, in collaboration with the patient client, a goal-specific treatment plan to increase physical functioning. They may be employed in hospitals, rehabilitation facilities, learning disability centers, or sports medicine facilities. Depending on their setting, their salaries range from $36,000 to $45,000 annually. Applicants for the 4- to 5-year kinesiotherapy education program require a high school diploma or equivalent (CAAHEP, 2011j).

Medical Assistant

Supervised by physicians, the **medical assistant** must have the ability to multitask. More than 60% of medical assistants work in medical offices and clinics. They perform both administrative and clinical duties. Medical assistants are employed by physicians more than any other allied health assistant. In 2006, their average entry-level salary was $27,000 per year. Their education consists of an associate's degree or a certificate or diploma program (CAAHEP, 2011k).

Medical Illustrator

Medical illustrators are trained artists that portray scientific information visually to teach both professionals and the public about medical issues. They work digitally or traditionally to create images of human anatomy and surgical procedures, as well as three-dimensional models and animations. Medical illustrators may be self-employed, work for pharmaceutical companies or advertising agencies, or be employed by medical schools. In 2006, annual salaries varied from $54,000 to $75,000. Applicants must have an undergraduate degree with a focus on art and premedical education. Their education program is 2 years and results in a master's degree (CAAHEP, 2011l).

Orthotist and Prosthetist

The **orthotist** and **prosthetist** specialists address neuromuscular/skeletal issues and develop a plan and a device to rectify any such issues. The orthotist develops devices called orthoses, or orthopedic appliances, used on the limbs and spines of individuals to increase function. The prosthetist designs "prostheses," or devices for patients who have limb amputations, to replace the limb function. Most of these allied health professionals work in hospitals, clinics, colleges, and medical schools. In 2006, their average annual salaries ranged from $42,000 to $60,000. Their education program consists of a 4-year program or a certificate program, which varies from 6 months to 2 years. Applicants for the 4-year program should have a high school diploma. Applicants for the certificate programs must have a 4-year degree (CAAHEP, 2011m).

Perfusionist

A **perfusionist** operates equipment to support or replace a patient's circulatory or respiratory function. Perfusion involves advanced life support techniques. Perfusionists may be responsible for administering blood by-products or anesthetic products during a surgical procedure. They may be employed by hospitals, surgeons, or group practices. Depending on experience, the average annual salary range is $60,000 to $100,000. The prerequisites for their education programs vary depending on the length of a program, which can range from 1 to 4 years depending on the individual's experience (CAAHEP, 2011n).

Personal Fitness Trainer

Personal fitness trainers are familiar with different forms of exercise. They have a variety of clients whom they serve one-on-one or in a group activity. They work with exercise science professionals or physiologists in corporate, clinical, commercial fitness, country club, or wellness centers. Employment of fitness workers is expected to increase 27% by 2016. In 2006, their average annual salary was $26,000. Their education programs consist of 1-year certificate or 2-year associate's degree programs. Applicants must have a high school diploma or equivalent for program entry (CAAHEP, 2011o).

Polysomnographic Technologist

Polysomnographic technologists perform sleep tests and work with physicians to provide diagnoses of sleep disorders. They monitor brain waves, eye movements, and other physiologic activity during sleep and analyze this information and provide it to the patient's physician. They work in sleep disorder centers that may be affiliated with a hospital or operate independently. In 2006, their average wages were $20 per hour. Applicants for their education programs should have a high school diploma or equivalent. Their education program ranges from a 2-year associate's degree to a 1-year certificate program (CAAHEP, 2011p).

Respiratory Therapist

Respiratory therapists—also known as respiratory care practitioners—evaluate, treat, and care for patients with breathing or other cardiopulmonary disorders. Practicing under the direction of a physician, respiratory therapists assume primary responsibility for all respiratory care therapeutic treatments and diagnostic procedures, including the supervision of respiratory therapy technicians. Respiratory therapists interview patients, perform limited physical examinations, and conduct diagnostic tests.

Hospitals account for the vast majority of job openings, but a growing number of openings will arise in other settings. An associate's degree is the minimum educational requirement, but a bachelor's or master's degree may be important for advancement. All states except Alaska and Hawaii require respiratory therapists to be licensed. An associate's degree is required to become a respiratory therapist. Training is offered at the postsecondary level by colleges and universities, medical schools, vocational-technical institutes, and the Armed Forces. Most programs award associate's or bachelor's degrees and prepare graduates for jobs as advanced respiratory therapists. According to the CAAHEP, 31 entry-level and 346 advanced respiratory therapy programs were accredited in the United States in 2008. About 81% of jobs were in hospitals, mainly in departments of respiratory care, anesthesiology, or pulmonary medicine. Much faster than average growth is projected for respiratory therapists. Job opportunities should be very good. The median annual wage of respiratory therapists was $52,200 in 2008 (Respiratory Care Therapist, 2011).

Specialists in Blood Bank Technology/Transfusion Medicine Specialist

Specialists in blood bank technology provide routine and specialized tests for blood donor centers, transfusion centers, laboratories, and research centers. Their average annual salaries range from $50,000 to $70,000. Applicants for their education programs must be certified in medical technology and have an undergraduate degree from an accredited educational institution. If they are not certified, they must have a degree from an accredited institution with a major in a biological or physical science and have appropriate work experience. This allied health education program ranges from 1 to 2 years (CAAHEP, 2011q).

Surgical Assistant

The **surgical assistant** is a specialized physician assistant. The main goal of the surgical assistant is to ensure the surgeon has a safe and sterile environment in which to perform surgery. The surgical assistant determines the appropriate equipment for a procedure, selects radiographs for the surgeon's reference, assists in moving the patient, confirms procedures with the surgeon, and assists with the procedure as directed by the surgeon. Their education programs range from 10 months to 22 months. In 2006, the average starting annual salary was $75,000. Applicants must have a bachelor of science or higher degree or an associate's degree in an allied health field with 3 years of recent experience, current CPR/basic life support certification, acceptable health and immunization records, and computer literacy (CAAHEP, 2011r).

Surgeon Technologist

Surgeon technologists are key team members of medical practitioners that provide surgery. They are responsible for preparing the operating room by equipping the room with the appropriate sterile supplies and verifying that the equipment is working properly. Prior to surgery, the surgeon technologist interacts with the patient to ensure the patient is comfortable, monitors the patient's vital signs, and reviews patient charts. During surgery, the surgeon technologist is responsible for ensuring that all surgery team members maintain a sterile environment and for providing instruments to the surgeon. Postsurgery, the surgeon technologist prepares the operating room for the next patient and may also provide follow-up care in the postoperative room. They work in hospitals, outpatient settings, or may be self-employed. Their average salary is $37,000 per year. Applicants for a surgeon technologist education program must have a high school diploma or equivalent. The programs range from 12 to 24 months (CAAHEP, 2011s).

Health Services Administrator

Health services administrators can be found at all levels of a healthcare organization. They manage hospitals, clinics, nursing homes, community health centers, and other healthcare facilities. At the top of the organization, they are responsible for strategic planning and the overall success of the organization. They are responsible for financial, clinical, and operational outcomes of an organization (Shi & Singh, 2008). Midlevel administrators also play a leadership role in departments and are responsible for managing their areas of responsibility. They may manage departments or individual programs. Administrators at all levels work with executive-level administration to achieve organizational goals. As healthcare costs continue to increase, it is important for health service administrators to focus on efficiency and effectiveness at all levels of management. Health services administration is taught at both the undergraduate and master's degree levels. The most common undergraduate degree is a degree in healthcare administration. Depending on the level of the administration position within an organization, a master's degree may be required. Undergraduate degrees may be acceptable for entry-level management positions. Salaries vary by administration level. Their average annual salary is $73,000 but varies depending on level of responsibility and size of the organization. Employment is expected to grow 16% by 2016. Approximately 40% of hospitals employ health services administrators. The most common master's degrees are the master of health services administration (MHA), master of business administration (MBA) with a healthcare emphasis, or a master of public health (MPH). The MHA or MBA degree provides a business-oriented education that health administrators need for managing healthcare organizations. However, an MPH degree provides insight into the importance of public health as an integral component of our healthcare system (BLS, 2011b).

Other Allied Health Professionals (Non–CAAHEP Accredited)

Radiation Therapist

Radiation therapy is used to treat cancer in the human body. As part of a medical radiation oncology team, **radiation therapists** use machines called linear accelerators to administer radiation treatment to patients. Radiation therapists work in hospitals or in cancer treatment centers. A bachelor's degree, associate's degree, or certificate in radiation therapy generally is required. Many states require radiation therapists to be licensed, and most employers require certification. With experience, therapists can advance to managerial positions. Employers usually require applicants to complete an associate's or a bachelor's degree program in radiation therapy. Individuals also may become qualified by completing an associate's or a bachelor's degree program in radiography, which is the study of radiological imaging, and then completing a 12-month certificate program in radiation therapy.

In 2009, there were 102 radiation therapy programs in the United States that were accredited by the American Registry of Radiologic Technologists. Employment is expected to increase much faster than the average, and job prospects should be good. Employment of radiation therapists is projected to grow by 27% between 2008 and 2018, which is much faster than the average for all occupations. The median annual wage of radiation therapists was $72,910 in 2008 (Radiation Therapists, 2012).

Nuclear Medicine Technologist

Nuclear medicine technologists administer radiopharmaceuticals to patients and then monitor the characteristics and functions of tissues or organs in which the drugs localize. Nuclear medicine technologists operate cameras that detect and map the radioactive drug in a patient's body to create diagnostic images. Nuclear medicine technology programs range in length from 1 to 4 years and lead to a certificate, an associate's degree, or a bachelor's degree. Many employers and an increasing number of states require certification or licensure. Aspiring nuclear medicine technologists should check the requirements of the state in which they plan to work. Generally, certificate programs are offered in hospitals, associate's degree programs in community colleges, and bachelor's degree programs in 4-year colleges and universities.

One-year certificate programs are typically for health professionals who already possess an associate's or bachelor's degree—especially radiologic technologists and diagnostic medical sonographers—but who wish to specialize in nuclear medicine.

The Joint Review Committee on Education Programs in Nuclear Medicine Technology accredits associate's and bachelor's degree training programs in nuclear medicine technology. In 2008, there were more than 100 accredited programs available. In spite of growth in nuclear medicine, the number of openings in the occupation each year will be relatively low. Job competition will be keen because the supply of properly trained nuclear medicine technologists is expected to exceed the number of job openings for technologists. The median annual wage of nuclear medicine technologists was $66,660 in 2008 (Nuclear Medicine Technologist, 2011).

Clinical Laboratory Technologist

Clinical laboratory testing plays a crucial role in the detection, diagnosis, and treatment of disease. **Clinical laboratory technologists**, also referred to as clinical laboratory scientists or medical technologists, and clinical laboratory technicians, also known as medical technicians or medical laboratory technicians, perform most of these tests. Clinical laboratory personnel examine and analyze body fluids and cells. They look for bacteria, parasites, and other microorganisms; analyze the chemical content of fluids; match blood for transfusions; and test for drug levels in the blood that show how a patient is responding to treatment. Clinical laboratory technologists generally require a bachelor's degree in medical technology or in one of the life sciences; clinical laboratory technicians usually need an associate's degree or a certificate. The usual requirement for an entry-level position as a clinical laboratory technologist is a bachelor's degree with a major in medical technology or in one of the life sciences; however, it is possible to qualify for some jobs with a combination of education and on-the-job and specialized training. The National Accrediting Agency for Clinical Laboratory Sciences (NAACLS) fully accredits about 479 programs for medical and clinical laboratory technologists, medical and clinical laboratory technicians, histo-technologists and histotechnicians, cytogenetic technologists, and diagnostic molecular scientists. NAACLS also approves about 60 programs in phlebotomy and clinical assisting. Rapid job growth and excellent job opportunities are expected. Most jobs will continue to be in hospitals, but employment will grow rapidly in other settings as well. Employment of clinical laboratory workers is expected to grow by 14% between 2008 and 2018, faster than the average for all occupations. The median annual wage of medical and clinical laboratory technologists was $53,500 in 2008 (Clinical Laboratory Technologists, 2011).

■ Conclusion

Healthcare personnel represent one of the largest labor forces in the United States. This chapter provided an overview of the different types of employees in the healthcare industry. Some of these positions require many years of education; however, others can be achieved through 1- to 2-year education programs. There are more than 200 occupations and professions among the more than 14 million healthcare workers in the United States (Sultz & Young, 2006). The healthcare industry will continue to progress as the U.S. trends in demographics, disease, and public health patterns change and as cost and efficiency issues, insurance issues, technological influences, and economic factors continue to evolve. More occupations and professions will develop as a result of these trends.

The major trend that will affect the healthcare industry is the aging of the U.S. population. The BLS predicts that half of the next decade's fastest growing jobs will be in the healthcare industry. Physician extenders and allied healthcare professionals will continue to play an increasing role in the provision of health care. This chapter contains information for the HR department in any healthcare organization that may be used to provide career education for employees. There were several career choices discussed in this chapter that may provide an opportunity for an existing employee to work in another department or organization. Organizations may provide education reimbursement for quality employees in return for an extended employment contract.

■ Vocabulary

Activities of daily living
Advanced practice nurse
Allied health professionals
Allopathic approach
Anesthesiologist assistant

Associate degree in nursing
Bachelor of science in nursing
Board certification
Cardiovascular technologist
Certified midwives

Certified nurse midwives
Certified nursing assistants
Chiropractors
Clinical laboratory technologist
Clinical psychologists
Counseling psychologists
Credentialing examination
Cytotechnologists
Dental assistants
Dental hygienists
Dentists
Diagnostic medical sonographer
Doctor of medicine
Doctor of osteopathic medicine
Electroneurodiagnostic
   technologist
Emergency medical technicians
Exercise physiologists
Exercise scientists
Experimental psychologists
Generalists
Health services administrator/
   manager
Hospitalist
Industrial-organizational
   psychologists
Kinesiotherapists
Licensed practical nurse

Medical assistant
Medical illustrator
Midlevel practitioners
National Practitioner Data Bank
Non-physician practitioner
Nuclear medicine technologist
Nurse practitioner
Optometrists
Orthotist
Perfusionists
Personal fitness trainer
Pharmacists
Physician assistant
Physician extenders
Podiatrists
Polysomnographic technologist
Prosthetist
Psychologists
Radiation therapists
Registered nurse
Research psychologists
Respiratory therapist
Social psychologists
Sonography
Specialists
Surgeon technologist
Surgical assistant
Transfusion medicine specialist

■ References

Allied Health Professions Overview (2012). Available at: http://explorehealthcareers.org/en/field/1/allied_health_professionals/eurl.axd/9f27a76084d7. Accessed September 23, 2011.

American Academy of Nurse Practitioners (2008). Available at: http://www.aanp.org/AANPCMS2/AboutAANP Accessed July 1, 2011.

American Podiatric Medical Association (2008). Available at: http://www.apma.org/MainMenu/AboutPodiatry/APMAOverview.aspx. Accessed July 1, 2011.

Association of Schools of Allied Health Professionals (2009). Available at: http://www.asahp.org/definition.htm. Accessed July 1, 2011.

BLS (2011a). Healthcare. Available at: http://www.bls.gov/oco/cg/cgs035.htm. Accessed January 14, 2011.

BLS (2011b). Chiropractors. Available at: http://www.bls.gov/oco/ocos071.htm. Accessed July 7, 2011.

BLS (2011c). Medical and health services managers. Available at: http://www.bls.gov/oco/ocos014.htm. Accessed July 7, 2011.

BLS (2011d). Optometrists. Available at: http://www.bls.gov/oco/ocos073.htm. Accessed July 7, 2011.

BLS (2011e). Pharmacists. Available at: http://www.bls.gov/oco/ocos079.htm. Accessed July 7, 2011.

BLS (2011f). Occupational employment and wages, chiropractors. Available at: www.bls.gov/oco/ocos097.htm. Accessed July 1, 2011.

BLS (2011g). Licensed practical and licensed vocational nurses. Available at: http://www.bls.gov/oco/ocos102.htm. Accessed July 1, 2011.

BLS (2011h). Occupational employment and wages, physician assistants. Available at: http://www.bls.gov/oes/2008/may/oes291071.htm. Accessed July 3, 2011.

BLS (2011i). Occupational employment and wages, pharmacists. Available at: http://bls.gov/oco/pdf/ocos079.pdf. Accessed December 11, 2011.

BLS (2011j). Occupational employment and wages, podiatrists. Available at: http://www.bls.gov/oes/2008/may/oes291081.htm. Accessed July 3, 2011.

BLS (2011k). Psychologists. Available at: http://www.bls.gov/oco/ocos056.htm. Accessed December 11, 2011.

BLS (2011l). Occupational employment and wages, registered nurses. Available at: http://www.bls.gov/oes/2008/may/oes291111.htm. Accessed July 3, 2011.

BLS (2011m). Clinical Laboratory Technologists. Available at: http://www.bls.gov/oco/pdf/ocos096.pdf. Accessed September 23, 2011.

Bradley, P. (2008). Nursing a Health Care Shortage. *Community College Weekly*. Available at: http://www.ccweek.com/news/templates/template.aspx?articleid=1439&zoneid=7. Accessed July 5, 2011.

Buchbinder, S. & Shanks, N. (2007). *Introduction to Health Care Management*. Sudbury, MA: Jones and Bartlett Publishers.

CAAHEP (2011a). Anesthesiologist assistant. Available at: http://www.caahep.org/Content.aspx?ID=20. Accessed Decemeber 11, , 2011.

CAAHEP (2011b). Cardiovascular technologist. Available at: http://www.caahep.org/Content.aspx?ID=21. Accessed December 11, 2011.

CAAHEP (2011c). Cytotechnology. Available at: http://www.caahep.org/Content.aspx?ID=22. Accessed December, 2011.

CAAHEP (2011d). Diagnostic medical sonography. Available at: http://www.caahep.org/Content.aspx?ID=23. Accessed December 11, 2011.

CAAHEP (2011e). Electroneurodiagnostic technology. Available at: http://www.caahep.org/Content.aspx?ID=38. Accessed December 11, 2011.

CAAHEP (2011f). Emergency medicine technician–paramedic. Available at: http://www.caahep.org/Content.aspx?ID=39. Accessed December 11, 2011.

CAAHEP (2011g). Exercise physiology. Available at: http://www.caahep.org/Content.aspx?ID=40. Accessed November 16, 2011.

CAAHEP (2011h). Exercise science. Available at: http://www.caahep.org/Content.aspx?ID=41. Accessed December 11, 2011.

CAAHEP (2011i). Kinesiotherapist. Available at: http://www.caahep.org/Content.aspx?ID=42. Accessed December 11, 2011.

CAAHEP (2011j). Medical assistant. Available at: http://www.caahep.org/Content.aspx?ID=43. Accessed December 11, 2011.

CAAHEP (2010k). Medical illustrators. Available at: http://www.caahep.org/Content.aspx?ID=44. Accessed December 11, 2011.

CAAHEP (2010l). Orthotist and prosthetist. Available at: http://www.caahep.org/Content.aspx?ID=45. Accessed December 11, 2011.

CAAHEP (2011m). Perfusionist. Available at: http://www.caahep.org/Content.aspx?ID=46. Accessed December 11, 2011.

CAAHEP (2011n). Personal fitness training. Available at: http://www.caahep.org/Content.aspx?ID=47. Accessed December 11, 2011.

CAAHEP (2011o). Polysomnographic technologist. Available at: http://www.caahep.org/Content.aspx?ID=48. Accessed December 11, 2011.

CAAHEP (2011p). Respiratory therapist. Available at: http://www.caahep.org/Content.aspx?ID=50. Accessed December 11 5, 2011.

CAAHEP (2011q). Specialist in blood banking technology/transfusion medicine. Available at: http://www.caahep.org/Content.aspx?ID=51. Accessed December 11, 2011.

CAAHEP (2011r). Surgical assisting. Available at: http://www.caahep.org/Content.aspx?ID=52. Accessed December 11, 2011.

CAAHEP (2011s). Surgical technologist. Available at: http://www.caahep.org/Content.aspx?ID=53. Accessed December 11, 2011.

National Center for Health Statistics (2008). *Health, United States, 2008, with Chartbook*. Washington, DC: U.S. Government Printing Office. Available at: http://www.cdc.gov/nchs/data/hus/hus08.pdf. Accessed July 1, 2011.

Nuclear Medicine Technologist (2011). Available at: http://www.bls.gov/oco/pdf/ocos104.pdf. Accessed September 23, 2011.

Pointer, D., Williams, S., Isaacs, S. & Knickman, J. (2008). *Introduction to Health Care*. New York, NY: John Wiley & Sons.

Radiation Therapists (2012). Available at: http://www.bls.gov/oco/pdf/ocos299.pdf. Accessed September 23, 2011.

Respiratory Care Therapist (2011). Available at: http://www.bls.gov/oco/pdf/ocos321.pdf. Accessed September 23, 2011.

Shi, L. & Singh, D. (2008). *An Introduction to Health Care in America: A Systems Approach*. Sudbury, MA: Jones and Bartlett Publishers.

Sultz, H. & Young, K. (2006). *Health Care USA*. Sudbury, MA: Jones and Bartlett Publishers.

Yordy, K. (2006). The nursing faculty shortage: Health care crisis. Available at: http://www.rwjf.org/files/publications/other/NursingFacultyShortage071006.pdf. Accessed July 7, 2011.

STUDENT WORKBOOK ACTIVITY 5.1

Complete the following case scenarios based on the information provided in the chapter. You must answer *in your own words*.

Real-Life Applications: Case Scenario 1

Because of the economic downturn, both you and your friend are now unemployed. You have heard that the healthcare industry is a growing industry for employment. You and your friend are unsure of the types of healthcare careers and whether you have the educational background to find a job in the healthcare industry. You have decided to become either a nurse or an allied health professional because there are so many opportunities. You and your friend decide to research these opportunities and share your results with each other.

Activity

You have chosen to explore two nursing jobs: licensed practical nurse and registered nurse. Your friend has narrowed the allied healthcare choices to three: physician assistant, cardiovascular technologist, and health services administrator. Provide (1) educational requirements, (2) job responsibilities, and (3) average wages for those careers in the spaces provided.

Nursing Options

Licensed practical nurse:

_____

_____

_____

_____

Registered nurse:

_____

_____

_____

_____

Allied Health Professionals

Physician assistant:

_____

_____

_____

_____

Cardiovascular technologist:

_____

_____

_____

_____

Health services administrator:

_____

_____

_____

_____

Real-Life Applications: Case Scenario 2

Your nephew cannot decide what type of physician he would like to be. He is currently in a premedical program, completing his undergraduate education. He is confused by whether he should pursue an MD degree or a DO degree. He asked you, an HR manager, to explain the difference between the two types of medical education.

Doctor of medicine:

_____

_____

_____

_____

Doctor of osteopathic medicine:

_____

_____

_____

_____

Real-Life Applications: Case Scenario 3

One of your employees approaches you about continuing her education. She has an undergraduate degree in science and mathematics. She decided to work for a few years in the healthcare industry before she continues her graduate education. She is interested in becoming an independent healthcare professional but is unsure of her direction. She has asked you for insight into this area of health care. You describe to her the many different options of pursuing a career in this category.

_____

_____

_____

_____

_____

Real-Life Applications: Case Scenario 4

After a disappointing career as a teacher, you have decided to enter the healthcare industry. You are unsure of what type of job you would like to pursue but want to be sure there is some accrediting body that provides guidance on different jobs. In your research, you continually encounter the acronym CAAHEP but are unsure of its significance.

Activity

Research the CAAHEP and discuss its importance to the healthcare industry.

Responses

_____

_____

_____

_____

_____

STUDENT WORKBOOK ACTIVITY 5.2

In Your Own Words

Please describe these core concepts in your own words.

Doctor of medicine:

_____

_____

_____

Doctor of osteopathic medicine:

_____

_____

_____

Allopathic approach:

_____

_____

_____

Exercise physiologist:

_____

_____

_____

Physician assistant:

_____

_____

_____

Medical illustrator:

_____

_____

_____

Kinesiotherapist:

_____

_____

_____

Pharmacist:

_____

_____

_____

Licensed vocational nurse:

_____

_____

_____

Certified midwife:

_____

_____

_____

Board certification:

_____

_____

_____

STUDENT WORKBOOK ACTIVITY 5.3

Internet Exercises

Write your answers in the spaces provided.

- Visit each of the websites listed in the text that follows.
- Name the organization.
- Locate its mission statement on its website. If the organization does not have a mission statement, describe its purpose.

- Provide a brief overview of the activities of the organization.
- Apply this organization to the chapter information.

Websites
http://www.aanp.org

Organization name:

_____

Mission statement:

_____

_____

_____

Overview of activities:

_____

_____

_____

Application to chapter information:

_____

_____

_____

http://www.apma.org

Organization name:

_____

Mission statement:

_____

_____

_____

Overview of activities:

_____

_____

_____

Application to chapter information:

_____

_____

_____

http://www.caahep.org

Organization name:

_____

Mission statement:

_____

_____

_____

Overview of activities:

_____

_____

_____

Application to chapter information:

_____

_____

_____

http://www.rwjf.org

Organization name:

_____

Mission statement:

_____

_____

_____

Overview of activities:

_____

_____

_____

Application to chapter information:

_____

_____

_____

http://bhpr.hrsa.gov
Organization name:

_____

Mission statement:

_____

_____

_____

Overview of activities:

_____

_____

_____

Application to chapter information:

_____

_____

_____

http://www.aapa.org
Organization name:

_____

Mission statement:

_____

_____

_____

Overview of activities:

_____

_____

_____

Application to chapter information:

_____

_____

_____

STUDENT ACTIVITY 5.4: DISCUSSION BOARDS FOR ONLINE, HYBRID, AND TRADITIONAL CLASSES

Discussion Board Guidelines

The discussion board is used in online courses in place of classroom lectures and discussion. The discussion board is the way in which students "link together" as a class. The following are guidelines to help focus on the discussion topic and to define the roles and responsibilities of the discussion coordinator and other members of the class. The educator will be the discussion moderator for this course.

1. The educator will post the discussion topic and directions for the upcoming week. These postings should all be responses to the original topic or responses to other students' responses. When people respond to what someone else has posted, they should start the posting with the person's name so it is clear which message they are responding to. **A response such as "Yes" or "I agree" does not count for credit. Your responses must be in your own words. You cannot copy and paste from the text.**

2. Postings (especially responses) should include enough information so the message is clear but should not be so long that it becomes difficult to follow. Remember, this is like talking to someone in a classroom setting.
3. Students should check the discussion daily to see if new information has been posted that requires their attention and response.

Good discussion will often include different points of view. Students should feel free to disagree or "challenge" others to support their positions or ideas. All discussion must be handled in a respectful manner. The following are suggested discussion boards for this chapter.

Discussion Boards

1. What is a hospitalist? Do you think a hospitalist has an important role in health care? Why or why not?
2. Describe the role of a physician assistant. Would you feel comfortable going to a physician assistant?
3. Discuss three employment-related pieces of legislation that you believe are very important and why.
4. Why is there a nursing shortage? What strategies can you suggest to rectify this employment issue?

Employee Benefits

The student will be able to:

- Describe six types of managed care organizations.
- List the four federally mandated employee benefits.
- Discuss the consumer-driven health plans.
- Evaluate long-term care insurance.
- Identify two types of disability insurance policies.
- Assess life insurance policies.

DID YOU KNOW THAT?

- A whole-life insurance policy provides permanent protection to the designated dependents.
- Women compose 70% of the labor workforce in the healthcare industry.
- "Cafeteria plans" are an example of flexible employee benefit plans, which enable employees to customize their benefit plans to satisfy their individual needs.
- A flexible work schedule is an alternative to a typical 40-hour, 9-to-5 work week and is becoming more popular in the healthcare industry.
- A nocturnist is a hospital physician who works only during night shifts.

■ Introduction

Different employee recruitment methods were previously described in this text. Employee benefits are a type of recruitment tool. There are benefits that are required by law, or mandatory benefits, which include social security, unemployment insurance, workers' compensation, and unpaid family and medical leave, and there are benefits that are not required by law, or voluntary benefits, such as health insurance, retirement plans, paid leave, and different types of family care. In addition to serving as a recruitment tool, benefits can also serve to retain and motivate employees. This chapter will describe employee benefits required by law and the optional employee benefits offered by organizations.

■ Social Security Act and Amendments

In 1935, President Franklin D. Roosevelt signed into law the Social Security Act, which created the Old Age, Survivors, and Disability Insurance (OASDI) program. In addition to several provisions for general welfare, the new act created a social insurance program designed to pay retired workers age 65 or older a continuing income after retirement. The 1939 amendments to the act made a fundamental change in the social security program. They added two new categories of benefits: payments to the spouse and minor children of a retired worker (so-called dependents benefits) and survivor's benefits paid to the family in the event of the premature death of a covered worker. This change transformed social security from a retirement program for workers into a *family-based* economic security program. The 1954 amendments to the act initiated a disability insurance program, which provided the public with additional coverage against economic insecurity. In the 1961 amendments to the act, the age at which men are first eligible for old-age insurance was lowered to 62 years, but with lower benefits (women previously were given this option in 1956). With the 1961 amendments to the Social Security Act, the Social Security Administration (SSA) became responsible for administering a new social insurance program, Medicare, for individuals age 65 years or older (History of the Social Security Administration, 2011).

In the 1970s, SSA became responsible for a new program, Supplemental Security Income (SSI). In the original **Social Security Act of 1935**, needy aged and blind individuals were covered, and, in 1950, the act began to cover needy disabled individuals. The federal government funds these three programs, or "adult categories," which are partially administered by state and local governments. In 1972, two important sets of amendments were enacted. These amendments created the SSI program and introduced automatic cost-of-living adjustments (COLAs) (Table 6.1). The bill creating the SSI program also contained important provisions for expanding the categories of social security beneficiaries, for instance to widows and widowers. It also provided a minimum retirement benefit and an adjustment to the benefit formula for early retirement at age 62 for men to make it consistent with that for women. It included an extension of Medicare to those who have received disability benefits for at least 2 years and to those with chronic renal disease. It also provided for delayed retirement credits to increase the benefits of those who delayed retirement until after age 65. Amendments passed in the 1980s and 1990s focused on streamlining the efficiency of social security programs. President Obama allocated

Table 6.1 Social Security Act (Old Age, Survivors, and Disability Insurance) and Amendments

1935	Social Security Act signed by President Roosevelt.
	Social insurance pension for individuals 65 years or older.
1939	Amendments included payments to spouses and minor children.
	Survivor's benefits to family of worker who has died.
1954	Amendments started a disability insurance program.
1961	Amendments lowered minimum age to 62 to collect pension.
	Medicare was established for those 65 years and older.
1972	Amendment established Supplemental Security Income.
	Cost of living adjustments for social security pensions.

$1 billion to the SSA to increase the efficiency of the system (History of the Social Security Administration, 2011).

Social security benefits are funded by a flat payroll tax on both employees and employers. Nearly 90% of U.S. employees are eligible for social security; however, railroad and government employees may have their own plans. Eligible employees will receive benefits based on earnings history and age at retirement. Early retirement is currently at age 62, but benefits are prorated. The full-retirement age varies based on year of birth. Table 6.2 outlines current retirement provisions based on an employee's age at retirement. According to the table, there have been different full-retirement ages. Age 65 years was mandated when the Social Security Act was passed. As years passed, the full-retirement age increased to the current age of 67 years. Table 6.2 also outlines how much a retirement pension would be reduced if an individual retired by age 62. For example, if an individual was born in 1960 or later and took an early retirement at age 62, the full-retirement monthly pension of $1,000 would be reduced 30% so that the individual would receive only $700 per month. A spouse's $500 survivor benefit would be reduced 35% so that the survivor would receive only $325 per month.

■ Unemployment Insurance

The Social Security Act of 1935 created the foundation for **unemployment insurance**. The Federal Unemployment Tax Act of 1939 (FUTA) provided the framework for what was established in the 1935 Act. FUTA requires employers and employees to pay a tax of 7.65% on employees' earnings on the first $102,000 of employee income: 6.2% goes to OASDI (decreased to 6% on July 1, 2011), and 1.45% goes to Medicare (Part A). Earnings over $102,000 are taxed only at the 1.45% Medicare rate

Table 6.2 Full-Retirement and Age 62 Benefits by Year of Birth

Year of Birth	Full (Usual) Retirement Age	At Age 62			
		A $1,000 Retirement Benefit Would Be Reduced To	The Retirement Benefit Is Reduced By	A $500 Spouse's Benefit Would Be Reduced To	The Spouse's Benefit Is Reduced By
1937 or earlier	65	$800	20.00%	$375	25.00%
1938	65 and 2 months	$791	20.83%	$370	25.83%
1939	65 and 4 months	$783	21.67%	$366	26.67%
1940	65 and 6 months	$775	22.50%	$362	27.50%
1941	65 and 8 months	$766	23.33%	$358	28.33%
1942	65 and 10 months	$758	24.17%	$354	29.17%
1943–1954	66	$750	25.00%	$350	30.00%
1955	66 and 2 months	$741	25.83%	$345	30.83%
1956	66 and 4 months	$733	26.67%	$341	31.67%
1957	66 and 6 months	$725	27.50%	$337	32.50%
1958	66 and 8 months	$716	28.33%	$333	33.33%
1959	66 and 10 months	$708	29.17%	$329	34.17%
1960 and later	67	$700	30.00%	$325	35.00%

*If you were born on January 1, you should refer to the previous year.
†If you were born on the first of the month, the benefit is figured as if your birthday was in the previous month. You must be at least 62 for the entire month to receive benefits.
‡Percentages are approximate due to rounding.
§The maximum benefit for the spouse is 50% of the benefit the worker would receive at full retirement age.

Source: http://www.socialsecurity.gov/retire2/agereduction.htm.

(What's New: FUTA, 2011). States are responsible for administering unemployment insurance programs. They have developed their own benefits programs, which typically last 26 weeks, but due to the economic recession and the subsequent American Recovery and Reinvestment Act of 2009, individuals may be qualified for up to 99 weeks of unemployment insurance. The average benefit is approximately 35% of the weekly wage of the individual. State rates vary depending on the **experience rating** of an employer, which means that states review how often an employer has used the unemployment program in the past. Employers who use the unemployment program will receive a higher tax rate. It is an incentive for employers to manage their employees to minimize layoffs (Noe et al., 2011). To receive benefits, employees (1) must be available for work during their period of unemployment, (2) must have worked at least four quarters, (3) must demonstrate they are actively seeking employment, and (4) must not have been terminated for poor performance or have quit.

States typically provide approximately 50% of the employee's earnings for a period of 26 weeks. However, because of the economic downturn, the federal government under its Emergency Unemployment Compensation program has extended the benefits to range from 34 to 53 weeks. If a state has very high unemployment, the unemployment benefits can be extended to 99 weeks (Office of Unemployment Insurance, 2011).

■ Workers' Compensation

The **workers' compensation** program protects both the employer and the employee if a job-related injury or illness occurs. Workers' compensation is a state program, so benefits vary by state. Employees are eligible for this program for the following issues: (1) medical care, (2) death, (3) disability, and (4) rehabilitation services. Most employees receive approximately 66⅔% of their earnings, which is tax-free. Workers' compensation programs are funded by the employer, who either contracts with a commercial insurer or self-insures. Depending on the industry and the risk of injury, rates can vary from 1% of the payroll to 100% of the payroll. Like unemployment insurance, rates can also vary based on the experience rating of the company (Noe et al., 2011).

These laws fall under **no-fault liability** or **no-fault insurance**, which were developed to avoid costly legal fees, and thus have no process to assess blame. The employee does not have to demonstrate that the employer was in the wrong, and the employer is protected from lawsuits unless it can be demonstrated that the employer was grossly negligent with respect to the working conditions (History of Workmen's Compensation, 2011). Unfortunately, there are disparities in how workers' compensation programs are implemented in each state. States often differ on the scope of permanent disability benefits and mental health coverage for any issues resulting from work. Experts estimate that 1 in 20 occupational disease victims receive workers' compensation benefits and 1 in 100 for occupational cancer. The American Public Health Association recommends that a national database be established on worker injuries, illnesses, toxic exposures, and diseases (APHA Policy: Workmen's Compensation Reform, 2009). As of this writing, workers' compensation is not reformed.

■ Family and Medical Leave

Because of the passage of the **Family and Medical Leave Act of 1993,** companies that have 50 or more employees are required to provide up to 12 weeks of unpaid projected job leave for a family issue such as birth, illness of self or family, or adoption. The act also covers the care of an employee's health problems that have affected job performance. A 2008 amendment offers an alternative option of 26 work weeks of leave to care for a member of the armed forces who is a spouse or close relative of the employee. Although the salary is not paid, the healthcare benefits continue (Family Medical and Leave Act, 2011). From a management perspective, it is difficult to lose an employee for 12 weeks; therefore, a plan should be in place to cover the responsibilities of the employee who will be on leave. An option to cross-train workers for the vacant position is a possibility, as is hiring a temporary worker to manage the workload.

■ Employee Optional Benefit Plans

There are other types of benefits that employers voluntarily offer and that often represent a recruitment tool for the organization. These types of **voluntary benefits** include medical insurance, paid time off, retirement plans, life insurance, disability insurance, long-term care insurance, childcare and eldercare, education reimbursement, and flexible work schedules—all optional benefits that can be very helpful to recruit and to retain employees.

Group Medical Insurance

Most employees and job seekers are concerned about receiving medical insurance because employer-sponsored health insurance is less expensive than individually purchased health insurance. Employers that offer health insurance must comply with the Consolidated Omnibus Budget Reconciliation Act of 1986 (COBRA), which requires employers to extend employees' health coverage for up to 3 years after a person leaves as a result of termination, after loss of full-time employee status, or upon the employee's death (spouse needs coverage) (Byars & Rue, 2006). The Patient Protection and Affordability Care Act of 2010 (PPACA) has put restrictions on health insurance companies from imposing lifetime or annual caps on health insurance reimbursement. The PPACA also assists those individuals who have been denied insurance because of preexisting conditions.

Comprehensive health insurance policies provide benefits that include outpatient and inpatient services, surgery, laboratory testing, medical equipment purchases, therapies, and other services such as mental health, rehabilitation, and prescription drugs. Most comprehensive policies have some exclusion attached to the policy. The opposite of comprehensive health insurance policies is **basic** or **major medical policies**, which reimburse hospital services such as surgeries and any expenses related to any hospitalization. There are limits on hospital stays. **Catastrophic health insurance policies** cover unusual illnesses with a high deductible and have lifetime reimbursement caps. There are also specific health insurance policies such as **disease-specific policies** for cancer, and so forth, and **Medigap policies** that provide supplemental insurance coverage for Medicare patients (Shi & Singh, 2008).

■ Types of Health Insurance Plans

There are two basic types of health insurance plans: **indemnity plans**, which are fee-for-service plans, and **managed care plans**, which include health maintenance organizations, preferred provider organizations, and point-of-service plans. Indemnity plans are contracts between a beneficiary and a health plan, but there is no contract between the health plan and providers. The beneficiary pays a premium to the health plan. When the beneficiary receives a healthcare service, the plan will reimburse the beneficiary an established fee for a particular service regardless of the provider's fees. The beneficiary will then reimburse the provider directly (Sultz & Young, 2006).

The managed care plan is a special type of health plan that focuses on cost containment of health services. The first type of managed care organization was the health maintenance organization, which evolved in the 1970s. As managed care organizations evolved, different types of managed care organizations developed. Managed care plans combine health services and health insurance functions to reduce administrative costs. For example, an employer contracts with a health plan for services on behalf of its employees. The employer is required to pay a set amount per enrolled employee on a monthly basis. The contracted health plan has a contract with certain providers to whom it pays on a monthly basis a fixed rate per member for services. Enrolled employees may share costs with a copayment. There is no deductible. The enrolled employees have restrictions on their choice of providers or incur larger copayments if they choose a provider out of the network. Many employers offer managed care plans because they are less expensive.

There are six organizational structures of managed care organization (MCOs):

1. **Health maintenance organizations** (HMOs): HMOs are the oldest type of managed care. Members must see their primary care provider first in order to see a

specialist. There are four types of HMOs: staff model, group model, network model, and the independent practice association.

- The **staff model** hires providers to work at a physical location.
- The **group model** negotiates with a group of physicians exclusively to perform services.
- The **network model** is similar to the group model, but these providers may see other patients who are not members of the HMO. There is a negotiated rate for service for members to see providers who belong to the network.
- The **independent practice associations** (IPAs) contract with a group of physicians who are in private practice to see MCO members at a prepaid rate per visit. The physicians may sign contracts with many HMOs. The physicians may also see non-HMO patients. This type of HMO was a result of the Health Maintenance Organization Act of 1973.

2. **Preferred provider organizations** (PPOs): These providers agree to a relative value-based fee schedule or a discounted fee to see members. They do not have a gatekeeper like the HMO, so a member does not need a referral to see a specialist. The PPO does not have a copay but does have a deductible. This plan was developed by providers and hospitals to ensure that nonmembers could still be served while a discount was still provided to MCOs for their members. A member may see a provider not in the network, but he or she may pay more out of pocket for the provider's services. The bill could be as much as 50% of the total bill. PPOs are currently the most popular type of plan (Sultz & Young, 2006; American Heart Association, 2011).

3. **Exclusive provider organizations** (EOPs): These organizations are similar to PPOs, but they restrict members to the list of preferred or exclusive providers that can be used.

4. **Physician hospital organizations** (PHOs): These organizations include physician hospitals, surgical centers, and other medical providers that contract with a managed care plan to provide health service (Judson & Harrison, 2006).

5. **Point-of-service (POS) plans:** The POS plans are a blend of the other MCOs—a type of HMO/PPO hybrid (American Heart Association, 2011). They encourage but do not require plan members to use a primary care provider who will become the gatekeeper of services. Members will receive lower fees if they use a gatekeeper model. Patients may see an out-of-network provider but are charged a higher rate. This type of plan was developed because of complaints about the inability of a member to choose his or her provider (Anderson, Rice & Kominski, 2007).

6. **Provider-sponsored organizations** (PSOs): These organizations are owned or controlled by healthcare providers. This emerging term describes provider organizations that are formed to contract directly with purchasers to deliver healthcare services. PSOs are formed by organizations such as IPAs. However, unlike IPAs, they assume insurance risk for their beneficiaries (Longest & Darr, 2008).

On-site Health Clinics: A recent trend in employee benefits that increases employees' wellness and reduces healthcare costs is the implementation of on-site medical healthcare clinics. The accessibility of these clinics increases the likelihood of employees not missing annual physical exams, obtaining prescriptions, and receiving routine preventive care such as mammograms, blood pressure screenings, and flu shots. Due to the cost of setting up a clinic, it is practical for companies that have at least 300 employees to implement this type of benefit (On-site Health Care Clinics, 2010). In 2010, 15% of large corporations had clinics providing primary-care services. Several smaller companies are sharing the cost of setting up joint on-site healthcare clinics (Cost Control, 2011).

Toyota Motor built an on-site medical center at its North American location in San Antonio. Although it cost $9 million to build, Toyota anticipates millions in healthcare cost savings. The on-site medical center has dramatically reduced the number of expensive referrals to specialists and emergency room visits. Productivity has increased because employees spend less time away from the job for a doctor's visit. Nissan, Harrah's Entertainment, Walt Disney Parks and Resorts, and Walgreens are now providng on-site health clinics (Welch, 2008).

Consumer-Driven Health Plans

A recent trend in health insurance plans is **consumer-driven health plans** (CDHPs), which are tax-advantaged plans with high deductible coverage. The most common CDHPs are **health reimbursement arrangements** (HRAs) and Health Savings Accounts (HSAs). HRAs or **personal care accounts** began in 2001 because of an Internal Revenue Service regulation. An HRA is funded by the employer but owned by the employees and remains with the company if the employee leaves. This has been an issue because the HRA has no portability (Wilensky, 2006).

An HSA, which was authorized by the Medicare Prescription Drug, Improvement, and Modernization Act of 2003, pairs high-deductible plans with fully portable employee-owned tax-advantaged accounts. This plan encourages consumers to become more cost-conscious when using the healthcare system because they are using their own funds for healthcare services. The HSA, unlike the HRA, is a portable account, which means it can be transferred to another employer when the employee changes jobs. HSAs encourage consumers to understand healthcare service pricing because these accounts are paired with a high deductible. America's Health Insurance Plans, an industry trade association, estimates that 4% of firms that offered benefits also offered an HSA or HRA (Wilensky, 2006).

Other types of CDHPs include **flexible spending accounts** (FSAs) and **medical savings accounts** (MSAs). FSAs provide employees with the option of setting aside pretax income to pay for out-of-pocket medical expenses. Employees must submit claims for these expenses, which are reimbursed from their spending accounts. The drawback is that the amount set aside must be spent within 1 year. Any unspent dollars cannot be rolled over, so it is very important to be very specific about the projected medical expenses.

Mandated as part of the Health Insurance Portability and Affordability Act of 1996, the MSA allows workers that are employed in firms with 50 or less employees and who have high-deductible health insurance plans to set aside pretax dollars to be used for healthcare premiums and nonreimbursed healthcare expenses (Buchbinder & Shanks, 2007).

Long-Term Care Insurance

As the life expectancy continues to increase in the United States, more people will require more healthcare services for chronic conditions. Unfortunately, Medicare and traditional health insurance policies do not pay for long-term care. Medicaid will pay for long-term care if individuals qualify for its program. **Long-term care insurance** was developed to cover services such as assistance with activities of daily living and care in an organizational setting. The cost of long-term care insurance can vary based on the type and amount of services selected, the age at time of purchase, and healthcare status. If an individual is already receiving long-term care or is in ill health, that individual may not qualify for long-term care insurance. Most long-term care insurance policies are comprehensive, which means they will cover expenses from home health care, hospice, respite care, assisted living, nursing homes, Alzheimer special care, and adult daycare centers. Long-term care policy costs vary greatly based on age and type of policy. The average annual premium for a policy purchased in 2007 by individual buyers of all ages was $2,200 (Buying LTC Insurance, 2011).

The **National Clearinghouse for Long Term Care** has provided the following information for purchasing long-term care insurance:

- The policyholder can select a daily benefit amount, which can range from $50 to $500 per day. The policyholder can select how much is paid on a daily basis, depending on the healthcare setting. The type of healthcare setting can also be identified such as home health care or skilled nursing facility.
- The policyholder can select a lifetime amount the policy will provide, which can range from $100,000 to $300,000. Policies that are more expensive will allow unlimited coverage with no dollar limit.
- The policyholder can also select an inflation option, which adjusts the coverage amount as one ages.
- Some policies may pay for family/friend long-term care for the policyholder. The policy may also provide reimbursement for equipment or transportation.

One hundred companies represent 15 insurers that offer long-term care. More employers are now offering long-term care insurance as an option to their employees. Employers do not contribute to the premium cost but may negotiate a better group rate. Long-term care insurance is becoming more popular because individuals are recognizing that their traditional health insurance and Medicare will not pay for long-term care (Buying LTC Insurance , 2011).

■ Life Insurance

Life insurance is frequently offered by employers. Employers purchase **life insurance** that will provide a sum to the beneficiaries, typically a spouse or dependent, upon the death of the employee. **Term life insurance** is the simplest type offered and the least expensive because there is no cash value attached to the policy. Employees offer basic term life insurance for all employees. It is valid through the period of employment. Employees can purchase additional or **supplemental term life insurance,** which increases the beneficiary amount for an additional premium. Depending on the insurance carrier, the employee may be required to submit a physical exam for the additional coverage. It is recommended that the employee purchase a policy valued at approximately two to five times his or her annual salary (Dratch, 2011). The biggest limitation on the policy is that it ends when the employment ends.

Whole-life insurance provides permanent protection to the dependents. The policy accrues a cash value. The premium for the policy is fixed during the lifetime of the policyholder and is guaranteed for life. The insurance company manages the cash that accrues in the policy, and the cash is tax deferred. The policyholder can cancel the policy when he or she no longer needs it.

Universal life insurance provides term coverage but also provides cash value with flexible premiums and schedules. The different types of life insurance are attractive optional benefits to those employees who have spouses or dependents (Fried & Fottler, 2008). Most employees expect dental and vision insurance as part of their basic health insurance package. **Dental insurance** is expensive with premiums rising annually. Basic dental insurance provides for cleaning of teeth every 6 months. There is less cost sharing for complicated dental procedures. **Vision coverage** often provides coverage for one annual eye exam and one pair of glasses or contact lenses. **Prescription drug benefits** are considered a good recruiting and retention tool for employees. They are expensive for the employer to offer but are necessary. As prescription drug costs rise, so will the premiums for this coverage. More programs are encouraging generic drug coverage rather than brand-name drug coverage. Some employers use **pharmacy benefit managers** (PBMs), which are companies that administer drug benefits for employers and health insurance carriers. They contract with managed care organizations, self-insured employers, Medicaid and Medicare managed care plans, federal health insurance programs, and local government organizations. Approximately 95% of all patients with drug coverage received benefits through a PBM. They manage approximately 70% of more than 3 billion prescriptions in the United States each year. The PBM integrates medical and pharmacy data of the population to determine which interventions are the most cost effective and clinically appropriate (Federal Trade Commission, 2011).

Long-term disability insurance is purchased by employees to ensure they will have income in the event of a disability. Disability insurance is offered to full-time permanent employees. It becomes active if an employee is unable to work for 90 to 180 days depending on the employer. The worker receives a percentage of his or her

Table 6.3 Top 10 Short-Term Disability Insurance Companies, Ranked by Earned Premium

Insurance Company	2007 Sales (in millions)
1. Hartford Life	$102.6
2. Lincoln Financial Group	$61.4
3. Unum	$60.7
4. Aetna	$42.6
5. Sun Life Financial	$41.7
6. MetLife	$40.9
7. CIGNA	$37.6
8. Reliance Standard	$36.8
9. Standard	$34.3
10. Prudential	$30.1

Source: Basics of Short-Term Disability (2011).

predisability salary. The disability pay is not taxed. Healthcare workers have more opportunities to become disabled because of the nature of their work environment. This particular benefit is often asked about by healthcare professionals when they are searching for employment (Fried & Fottler, 2008). **Short-term disability benefits** pay a portion of one's salary, approximately 40% to 65%, if one becomes temporarily disabled because of injury or sickness. These benefits last 3 to 6 months. The average 2009 group premium per year was approximately $210. Table 6.3 itemizes the top insurance companies that provide short-term disability benefits.

Short-term disability insurance may be a viable option for healthcare workers. According to the Council for Disability Awareness, 3 in 10 individuals entering the workforce will experience a disability before retiring (Basics of Short-Term Disability, 2011).

■ Retirement Plans

When individuals are searching for jobs, they are concerned with their healthcare benefits and what type of retirement plans are offered. Retirement plans represent a benefit for past work performed in the organization. There are basic retirement plans: private pension plans, defined benefit plans, and defined contribution plans. Although most people receive social security as a pension, the amount is not sufficient, so retirement plans are of interest to potential employees. In **contributory**

retirement plans, funds are contributed by both employers and employees, whereas in **noncontributory retirement plans,** all funds are contributed only by the employers. Noncontributory plans are unusual because most employers can no longer afford to offer these types of plans. These types of plans are common in government organizations. Funds are accrued in a **defined benefit plan** by the employer, which guarantees that it will invest a designated amount each year, so that when an employee retires, he or she is guaranteed a specified annual income, which is determined by service time, earnings, and age. These types of plans encourage employees to remain with the organization for a long period, reducing voluntary turnover. These types of plans are guaranteed by the Employee Retirement Income Security Act of 1974 (ERISA), which mandates that organizations must protect their retirees, establish **vesting rights,** and establish portability rules. Vesting occurs when an employee leaves an organization prior to retirement and is entitled to receive the funds that were accruing in his or her retirement or pension fund. **Portability** enables employees to move retirement funds if they move to another job. The **Pension Benefit Guarantee Corporation** (PBGC) was created by ERISA as the federal agency that insures retirement benefits and guarantees a basic benefit if the employer has financial difficulties. Employers must contribute a specified amount per employee to the PBGC. According to its website, the PBGC protects the retirement incomes of more than 44 million American workers in more than 27,500 private-sector–defined benefit pension plans. PBGC pays for monthly retirement benefits, up to a guaranteed maximum, for nearly 801,000 retirees in 4,200 single-employer and multiemployer pension plans that cannot pay promised benefits. Including those who have not yet retired and participants in multiemployer plans receiving financial assistance, PBGC is responsible for the current and future pensions of about 1.5 million people (PBGC, 2011). The PBGC has been utilized very frequently during the U.S. economic recession.

A **defined contribution plan** is an individual account for each employee, which specifies the size of the investment into the account. The retirement benefit is determined by the performance of the account. A **401(k) plan** is a typical defined contribution plan. Employees contribute a percentage of their earnings, which employers match. There is a limit to the amount of contributions each year.

■ Other Benefits

Paid Vacation and Sick Leave

Most companies provide days off for major holidays such as Christmas and New Year's Day, Thanksgiving, Fourth of July, Labor Day, and Memorial Day. In the healthcare industry, depending on the type of organization, many employees must work on these holidays, but they receive extra compensation for working. Employees are eligible for paid time off such as **paid vacation leave** once they work for the organization for a period of time, typically a year. Employees will also be eligible for **paid sick leave,** which is accrued hourly each month. Sick leave varies by organization. Some organizations require **sick leave** to be used in one calendar year. Other organizations allow employees to roll over sick leave up to a maximum number of hours. In addition, when a person retires, he or she is compensated for the number of sick hours that are in his or her account. Some organizations do not differentiate between vacation and sick leave. Employees accrue **paid time off** (PTO), which functions in the same manner as paid vacation and sick leave, but the employee does not inform the organization why he or she is taking time off. The concept of paid time off can be an incentive for employees because they do not have to differentiate between vacation and actual sick leave. However, a PTO system needs policies in place to ensure it is not abused. Most employees who have a traditional vacation and sick leave program rarely take all of their sick leave in one year. However, with a PTO program, the employees will use all of their paid time off, resulting in increased time off from the organization (Reh, 2011).

Childcare and Eldercare

The percentage of women in the workforce has increased since 1970. In 2008, the overall labor rate of mothers with children younger than 18 years was 71% compared with 94% of fathers. The labor rate of mothers with children under 3 years of age was 59%. In 2008, there were nearly 10 million single-parent mothers with children under 18 years of age in the United States. Of those 10 million, 71% were employed. There were 1.8 million single-parent fathers with children under 18 years. Of those 1.8 million, approximately 80% were employed. There were 2 million single-parent mothers with children under 3 years of age; of those 2 million, 57% were employed. There were 232,000 single-parent fathers with children under 3 years of age, with 77% of those 232,000 employed (Working Parents, 2011). These demographics have resulted in an increased need by employers to offer **childcare services** as an optional employee benefit. In addition to these general labor statistics, nurse positions are typically held by females. Approximately 75% of healthcare positions are held by females in the areas of nursing midwifery and community health workers (WHO, 2008). Typically, industries that require 24-hour workers offer some type of childcare services. Annually, *Fortune* magazine publishes a list of the top 100 best companies for employment. Results indicate that nearly 25% of the companies on the list provide on-site childcare, and many of these companies are in the healthcare industry (100 Best Companies to Work For, 2011). Statistics have also indicated that with the increased life expectancy of the U.S. population, there has been increased pressure on children to manage the need to care for their aging parents.

A recent survey indicated that U.S. businesses lose $33.6 billion annually due to absenteeism, workday interruptions, and employee turnover caused by aging relative issues. More companies are assisting employees with **eldercare** such as by providing training, offering consultants for eldercare services, and allowing employees to use their sick leave to take care of their parents. **Dependent care accounts**, which allow workers to set aside $5,000 for caregiver costs and typically include childcare, are now including eldercare (Kotz, 2006).

Education Reimbursement

Many companies offer reimbursement for all levels of education. A company is more likely to provide **education reimbursement** opportunities if the program increases the training and skills of an employee to the advantage of the company. This type of benefit can be an excellent tool for motivation and retention of quality employees. Healthcare employers often offer reimbursement for education that would increase the employee's contribution to the organization such as by providing tuition reimbursement for licensed practical nurses to attain their registered nurse degree (Swenson, 2010). The federal government recognizes the benefit of providing tuition reimbursement and allows employers to reimburse $5,250 tax-free to each qualified employee. Employers will offer guidelines for this reimbursement such as by offering it to full-time employees only or by stipulating additional years of employment of the employee if his or her tuition is reimbursed (Adkins, 2010).

Flexible Work Schedules

A **flexible work schedule** is an alternative to a typical 40-hour, 9-to-5 work week. The Fair Labor Standards Act does not address flexible work schedules, so it is the responsibility of the employer to establish guidelines for this type of work schedule. Flexible work schedules are becoming typical in the healthcare industry because 24-hour care may be needed in different types of healthcare facilities such as hospitals and skilled nursing facilities. With a disproportionate percentage of female employees in the healthcare industry who are main caregivers, flexible work schedules are an option to recruit and retain quality employees. A 2009 employee benefits report found that of those healthcare workers who resigned, 72% quit because the hours did not accommodate family and social time. For example, Baptist Memorial Health Care Corporation, located in Tennessee, surveyed its employees to determine their work schedule preferences. The nurses preferred weekend-only schedules or floating schedules. Because of the change, patient satisfaction increased, and turnover rates declined. Bryan LGH Medical Center in Nebraska opted to hire **nocturnists,** who are hospitalists that only work the night shift as their preference. This allowed daytime physicians to manage their day schedule. Chilton Memorial Hospital in New Jersey opted for telecommuting of its data-entry employees after the implementation of its electronic medical record system, which resulted in increased employee satisfaction (Howell, 2010).

■ Selecting Employee Benefits

As discussed earlier, there are certain employee benefits that must be legally offered; however, employers have great freedom to select other types of benefits. Employers must assess what competitors are offering and what the industry is offering because employees have a level of expectation as to what type of benefits they will be provided. Most employees expect medical insurance with vision and dental benefits. This type of information is available from the Bureau of Labor Statistics, from their annual **Employee Benefits Survey (EBS)**. The EBS targets approximately 6,000 private and government employers to determine what type of benefits are commonly provided. The employers are categorized by size of establishment and type of industry. According to 2011 EBS results, 91% of full-time workers in private industry were offered paid vacation benefits, but only 37% of part-time workers received this benefit. Paid sick leave was offered to 75% of full-time workers, but only 25% of part-time workers received this benefit. Nearly 65% of private industry workers had access to retirement benefits; however, nearly 90% of government workers had this benefit available to them (Employee Benefits in the U.S., 2011). These data indicate that full-time government workers receive more benefits than full-time private industry workers do; however, the salary and wages of private industry workers are often higher than those of government workers.

The EBS information is an excellent resource for both private and government employers; however, surveying employees for benefit preferences would be an excellent option because the demographic makeup of the company may differ from that of secondary data sources.

■ Cafeteria Plans

"Cafeteria plans" are employee benefits plans that provide flexibility to employees with different benefits needs. These types of plans offer alternative benefits that employees can choose, and they can decide the amount of the benefit. A typical cafeteria plan allows a monetary budget for each employee that can be spent on his or her chosen benefits. An advantage to offering this type of plan is the ability for the employee to customize his or her benefits plan. Examples of alternative benefits would be child or parent daycare, education reimbursement, or a health facility membership The disadvantage to a cafeteria plan is the high administrative cost. However, there are software packages that have alleviated this issue. Companies may also opt to select a third-party administrator such as **eflexgroup** to manage a cafeteria plan. Although a cafeteria health plan can be very attractive to potential employees, it is important that the company perform a cost–benefit analysis to determine administrative costs (FAQs about Cafeteria Plans, 2011).

■ Conclusion

There are four legally mandated employee benefits: social security, unemployment insurance, workers' compensation, and family and medical leave. However, there are several employee benefits that employers can offer to employees that can be used as a recruitment and/or retention tool. Employees expect employers to provide medical insurance including dental and vision plans, vacation and sick leave, and retirement plans. However, employers have the opportunity to offer other benefits such as education reimbursement, childcare or eldercare services, or flexible work schedules. Employers may consider a cafeteria plan, which enables employees to select which benefits are best suited for their lifestyles. Employers should survey their employees and their competition to determine the best type of benefits package that would motivate and retain quality employees. Establishing a quality benefits package would also be an excellent recruitment tool. The human resources (HR) department plays an important role in educating employees about their different benefits. Although most organizations provide an orientation to new employees that reviews benefits and also provide an employee benefit handbook, benefit education is ongoing in an organization. Often, HR departments will invite experts about disability and long-term care insurance to the organization to provide information to employees about their benefits choices.

■ Vocabulary

401(k) plan
Basic medical policies
Cafeteria plans
Catastrophic health insurance
    policies
Childcare services
Comprehensive health insurance
    policies
Consumer-driven health plans
Contributory retirement plans
Dependent care accounts
Defined benefit plan
Defined contribution plan
Dental insurance
Disease-specific policies
Education reimbursement
eflexgroup
Employee benefits survey (EBS)

Eldercare services
Exclusive provider organizations
Experience rating
Family and Medical Leave Act of
    1993
Flexible spending accounts
Flexible work schedules
Group model
Health maintenance organizations
Health reimbursement arrangements
Indemnity plans
Independent practice associations
Life insurance
Long-term care insurance
Long-term disability insurance
Major medical policies
Managed care plans
Medical saving accounts

Medigap policies
National Clearinghouse for Long Term Care
Network model
Nocturnists
No-fault insurance
No-fault liability
Noncontributory retirement plans
Paid sick leave
Paid time off
Paid vacation leave
Pension Benefit Guarantee Corporation
Personal care accounts
Pharmacy benefit managers
Physician hospital organizations
Point-of-service plans

Portability
Preferred provider organizations
Prescription drug benefits
Provider-sponsored organizations
Short-term disability benefits
Short-term disability insurance
Social Security Act of 1935
Staff model
Supplemental term life insurance
Term life insurance
Unemployment insurance
Universal life insurance
Vesting rights
Vision coverage
Voluntary benefits
Whole-life insurance
Workers' compensation

■ References

Adkins, M. (2010). Employee tuition reimbursement policy. Available at: http://www.ehow.com/about_6595400_employee-tuition-reimbursement-policy.html. Accessed July 31, 2011.

American Heart Association (2011). Managed health care plans. Available at: http://www.americanheart.org/presenter.jhtml?identifier=4663. Accessed July 15, 2011.

Anderson, R., Rice, T. & Kominski, G. (2007). *Changing the U.S. Health Care System*. San Francisco, CA: Jossey-Bass.

APHA Policy: Workmen's Compensation Reform (2009). Available at: http://www.apha.org/NR/rdonlyres/B240302E-94EF-4456-966F-6AEF329C289E/0/WorkersCompDraftNov102009.pdf. Accessed January 25, 2011.

Basics of Short-Term Disability (2011). Available at: http://www.insure.com/articles/disabilityinsurance/short-term-disability.html. Accessed January 24, 2011.

Buchbinder, S. & Shanks, N. (2007). *Introduction to Health Care Management*. Sudbury, MA: Jones and Bartlett Publishers.

Buying LTC Insurance (2011). Available at: http://longtermcare.gov/LTC/Main_Site/Paying/Private_Financing/LTC_Insurance/Buying.aspx. Accessed December 13, 2011.

Byars, L. & Rue, L. (2006). *Human Resource Management* (8th ed.). New York, NY: McGraw-Hill/Irwin, pp. 371–383.

Cost Control: Companies Expand Workplace Clinics (2011). Available at: http://www.thefiscaltimes.com/Articles/2011/05/27/Cost-Control-Companies-Expand-Workplace-Clinics.aspx#page1. Accessed December 13, 2011.

Dratch, D. (2011). Major types of life insurance. Available at: http://www.bankrate.com/brm/news/insur/20020917b.asp. Accessed January 24, 2011.

Employee Benefits in the U.S. (March 2011). Available at: http://www.bls.gov/news.release/ebs2.nr0.htm. Accessed December 13, 2011.

Family Medical Leave Act (2011). Available at: http://www.dol.gov/whd/fmla/. Accessed January 23, 2011.

FAQs about Cafeteria Plans (2011). Available at: http://www.irs.gov/govt/fslg/article/0,,id=112720,00 .html#1. Accessed July 11, 2012.

Federal Trade Commission (2011). Available at: http://www.www.ftc.gov/opa/2004/07/healthcarept .shtm. Accessed July 15, 2011.

Fried, B. & Fottler, M. (2008). *Human Resources in Healthcare* (3rd ed.). Chicago, IL: Health Administration Press, pp. 443–449.

History of the Social Security Administration (2011). Available at: http://www.ssa.gov/history/ briefhistory3.html. Accessed July 12, 2011.

History of Workmen's Compensation (2011). Available at: http://www.iaiabc.org/i4a/pages/index .cfm?pageid=3299. Accessed January 23, 2011.

Howell, W. (2010). Hospitals offer flexible work schedules to boost morale, productivity. Available at: http://www.hhnmag.com/hhnmag_app/jsp/articledisplay.jsp?dcrpath=HHNMAG/Article/ data/08AUG2010/1008HHN_Inbox_workforce&domain=HHNMAG. Accessed December 13, 2011.

Judson, K. & Harrison, C. (2006). *Law & Ethics for Medical Careers*. New York, NY: McGraw-Hill.

Kotz, D. (2006). Need help? Ask your employer. Available at: http://health.usnews.com/usnews/health/ articles/061119/27benefit.htm. Accessed February 5, 2011.

Longest, B., Jr. & Darr, K. (2008). *Managing Health Services Organizations and Systems*. Baltimore, MD: Health Professions Press.

Noe, R., Hollenbeck, J., Gerhart, B. & Wright, P. (2011). *Fundamentals of Human Resource Management* (3rd ed.). New York, NY: McGraw-Hill/Irwin, pp. 388–389.

Office of Unemployment Insurance (2011). Available at: http://workforcesecurity.doleta.gov/unemploy/ claims_arch.asp. Accessed January 25, 2011.

100 Best Companies to Work For (2011). Available at: http://money.cnn.com/magazines/fortune/ bestcompanies/2011/benefits/index.html. Accessed February 5, 2011.

On-site Health Care Clinics Gain in Popularity (2010). Available at: http://www.mjinsurance.com/ news-and-events/archived-posts/on-site-health-care-clinics-gain-in-popularity.aspx. Accessed December 13, 2011.

The Pension Benefit Guaranty Corporation (2011). Who we are. Available at: http://www.pbgc.gov/ about/who-we-are.html. Accessed December 13, 2011.

Reh, J. (2011). Sick Leave vs. Paid Time Off (PTO). Available at: http://management.about.com/od/ conflictres/a/SickLvPTO1104.htm. Accessed December 13, 2011.

Shi, L. & Singh, D. (2008). *An Introduction to Health Care in America: A Systems Approach*. Sudbury, MA: Jones and Bartlett Publishers.

Sultz, H. & Young, K. (2006). *Health Care USA*. Sudbury, MA: Jones and Bartlett Publishers.

Swenson, P. (2010). Why employers offer tuition reimbursement. Available at: http://www.ehow .com/about_6549096_employers-offer-tuition-reimbursement.html. Accessed February 7, 2011.

Welch, D. (2008). Health-Care Reform, Corporate Style. Available at: http://www.businessweek.com/ print/magazine/content/08_32/b4095000246100.htm. Accessed December 13, 2011.

What's New: FUTA (2011). Available at: http://www.irs.gov/instructions/i940/ar01.html. Accessed January 25, 2011.

WHO (2008). Spotlight on statistics: A fact file on workforce healthcare statistics. Available at: http://www.who.int/hrh/statistics/spotlight2/en/index.html. Accessed February 4, 2011.

Wilensky, G. (2006). Consumer driven health plans. Early evidence and potential impact on hospitals. *Health Affairs*, 25(1):174–186.

Working parents (2011). Available at: http://www.catalyst.org/publication/252/working-parents. Accessed February 5, 2011.

STUDENT WORKBOOK ACTIVITY 6.1

Complete the following case scenarios based on the information provided in this chapter. Your responses must be *in your own words*.

Real-Life Applications: Case Scenario 1

The HR manager has discovered that the high turnover rate of the nurses and physicians in your organization is due to the inflexibility of the scheduling, not allowing for lifestyle and family issues. She has asked for a benefit plan that would reduce the turnover.

Activity

Outline a specific plan that would address the inflexibility of the scheduling of the nurses and physicians.

Responses

_____

_____

_____

_____

Real-Life Applications: Case Scenario 2

You are responsible for explaining the mandated employee benefits offered by the organization to newly hired employees.

Activity

Explain the four different mandated employee benefits as stipulated by federal law. Be sure to include any employee contributions to these benefits.

Responses

_____

_____

_____

_____

Real-Life Applications: Case Scenario 3

ABC Hospital Care has just hired you as a nurse manager. As part of your responsibilities, you are responsible for providing assistance to new nurse hires on their selection of medical insurance. They are newly graduated from nursing school and have never worked before and are unsure of what type of medical insurance they should select.

Activity

Explain the difference between an indemnity plan and a managed care plan. Describe four different managed care programs that are being offered by your employer.

Responses

_____

_____

_____

_____

Real-Life Applications: Case Scenario 4

The skilled nursing facility you work for has just hired two older nurses. They have approached you because you have worked there for 10 years and have asked you to explain what type of benefits are offered for older employees.

Activity

Explain the different disability insurance options and discuss the pros and cons of long-term care insurance.

Responses

_____

_____

_____

_____

STUDENT WORKBOOK ACTIVITY 6.2

In Your Own Words

Please describe these core concepts in your own words.

Indemnity plan:

_____

_____

_____

_____

Flexible work schedules:

_____

_____

_____

_____

Experience rating:

_____

_____

_____

_____

No-fault insurance:

_____

_____

_____

_____

Pharmacy benefit managers:

_____

_____

_____

_____

Vesting rights:

_____

_____

_____

_____

Portability:

_____

_____

_____

_____

Pension Benefit Guarantee Corporation:

_____

_____

_____

_____

Term life insurance:

_____

_____

_____

_____

STUDENT WORKBOOK ACTIVITY 6.3

Internet Exercises

Write your answers in the spaces provided.

- Visit each of the websites that are listed in the text that follows.
- Name the organization.
- Locate its mission statement on its website. If the organization does not have a mission statement, describe its purpose.
- Provide a brief overview of the activities of the organization.
- Apply this organization to the chapter information.

Websites

http://www.apha.org

Organization name:

_____

Mission statement:

_____

_____

_____

Overview of activities:

_____

_____

_____

Application to chapter information:

_____

_____

_____

http://www.ssa.gov

Organization name:

_____

Mission statement:

_____

_____

_____

Overview of activities:

_____

_____

_____

Application to chapter information:

_____

_____

_____

http://www.hhnmag.com
Organization name:

_____

Mission statement:

_____

_____

_____

Overview of activities:

_____

_____

_____

Application to chapter information:

_____

_____

_____

http://www.eflexgroup.com

Organization name:

_____

Mission statement:

_____

_____

_____

Overview of activities:

_____

_____

_____

Application to chapter information:

_____

_____

_____

http://www.catalyst.org
Organization name:

_____

Mission statement:

_____

_____

_____

Overview of activities:

_____

_____

_____

Application to chapter information:

_____

_____

_____

http://www.pbgc.gov
Organization name:

_____

Mission statement:

_____

_____

_____

Overview of activities:

_____

_____

_____

Application to chapter information:

_____

_____

_____

STUDENT ACTIVITY 6.4: DISCUSSION BOARDS FOR ONLINE, HYBRID, AND TRADITIONAL ONGROUND CLASSES

Discussion Board Guidelines

The discussion board is used in online courses in place of classroom lectures and discussion. The discussion board is the way in which students "link together" as a class. The following are guidelines to help focus on the discussion topic and to define the roles and responsibilities of the discussion coordinator and other members of the class. The educator will be the discussion moderator for this course.

1. The educator will post the discussion topic and directions for the upcoming week. These postings should all be responses to the original topic or responses to other students' responses. When people respond to what someone else has posted, they should start the posting with the person's name so it is clear which message they are responding to. **A response such as "Yes" or "I agree" does**

not count for credit. **Your responses must be in your own words. You cannot copy and paste from the text.**

2. Postings (especially responses) should include enough information so the message is clear but should not be so long that it becomes difficult to follow. Remember, this is like talking to someone in a classroom setting.

3. Students should check the discussion daily to see if new information has been posted that requires their attention and response.

Good discussion will often include different points of view. Students should feel free to disagree or "challenge" others to support their positions or ideas. All discussion must be handled in a respectful manner. The following are suggested discussion boards for this chapter.

Discussion Boards

1. Why was managed care developed? Do you think managed care is a good way to provide healthcare services? Why or why not?

2. What is the difference between an HMO and a PPO? Which one do you prefer? Research the Internet to find one HMO and one PPO.

3. What is long-term care insurance? Do you think this is a useful tool? Would you buy it?

4. What are cafeteria plans? What is one advantage and one disadvantage to these plans? Would you want to participate in this type of healthcare plan?

Training, Developing, and Motivating Healthcare Employees

The student will be able to:

- Compare the difference between training and professional development programs.
- Describe an organizational and personnel needs assessment.
- Discuss five types of employee training.
- Compare the difference between intrinsic and extrinsic rewards.
- Assess three motivational theories as they apply to health care.
- Evaluate three motivational strategies as they apply to health care.

DID YOU KNOW THAT?

- On-the-job training is an excellent method of learning a job.
- Internships are types of on-the-job training.
- Webinars are web-based seminars that offer employee training.
- Virtual reality is used to practice surgery.
- Motivation is composed of the ability of the employee to perform the work and a work environment that encourages employee performance.

■ Introduction

The goal of healthcare organizations is to provide quality care to their patients. Nurses, physicians, and other healthcare providers have direct contact with patients. There are also different types of healthcare employees that provide indirect care to patients. Laboratory technologists and technicians have a major role in diagnosing disease, assessing the impact of interventions, and applying highly technical procedures, but they may never see the patients directly.

Regardless of their roles, employees that underperform could risk the lives of their patients. Research on high-performing organizations, including healthcare organizations, reveals that employees are motivated to perform well by the quality of the work environment. A quality work environment includes initiatives such as employee empowerment, training and career development programs, pay for performance, management transparency and support, and work–life balance (Lowe, 2002). This chapter will describe different motivational theories and different organizational strategies to motivate employees to perform.

■ How to Motivate Employees

What Is Motivation?

Motivation is composed of two major factors: the ability of the employee to perform well and a work environment that encourages the employee's performance. If an organization has a quality selection process in place that will lead to hiring of employees with the appropriate knowledge, skills, and abilities (KSAs), the second component of motivation is the processes that the organization has established to motivate an employee's performance. According to Hitt, Miller, and Colella (2006), employee performance is a combination of ability and motivation. Two employees may have the same ability, but their performance may differ because they are motivated by different forces. In order for an employee to be motivated, the employee must view the process or environment as a reward that he or she values. Motivational theorists have analyzed several theories over the past 100 years to explain employee performance differences.

Motivational Theories

Employee rewards can be extrinsic or intrinsic. **Extrinsic** or **external rewards** are outcomes that have been developed by the organization that encourage high performance. An employee is motivated by the possibility of achieving a bonus or a promotion. **Intrinsic** or **internal rewards** are the positive feelings of employees that are the result of an action such as performing a job well (Knicki & Kreitner, 2009). An employee experiences a positive emotional experience because of his or her positive job performance. Regardless of whether an employee is motivated by either intrinsic or extrinsic rewards, the employee should receive recognition. To ensure that the rewards are valued by employees, the human resources (HR) department should survey employees to assess preference.

There are several motivational theories that have been discussed over the past decades. Four theories will be explored: expectancy theory, equity theory, goal-setting theory, and a four-prong model of intrinsic motivation. They focus on how employees' feelings or emotions influence their performance. **Expectancy theory** states that motivation is a function of an employee's expectation that his or her efforts will lead to a certain level of performance. If an employee works overtime to care for a patient or a laboratory technician works overtime to analyze emergency test results, the employee would expect praise from his or her supervisor and possible overtime pay. As part of expectancy theory, the concept of valence of value is addressed. Any outcome must be considered valuable or have **valence** to an employee or the outcome will not be a motivator.

Equity theory focuses on employer fairness. Employees expect to be paid fairly in comparison with other employees in the same position and to receive the same rewards if both employees work similarly. If protected class employees are not treated fairly, legality issues of discrimination can result. Equity theory is important in healthcare because of the continued nursing shortage, which creates unequal staffing levels and job dissatisfaction. This is particularly true in hospital settings because there is a higher patient to nurse ratio, which results in emotional exhaustion (Aiken, Clarke, Sloane, Sochalski & Silber, 2002).

Goal-setting theory states that establishing performance goals for employees encourages employee performance. Setting challenging and specific goals that are realistic to obtain are a motivator for high performance. Employee participation in goal setting may also have a positive impact on job performance (Hitt, Miller & Colella, 2006; Buchbinder & Shanks, 2007).

Thomas (2000) developed a four-prong model of intrinsic motivation: sense of choice, competence, meaningfulness, and progress. A **sense of choice** is the opportunity an employee feels when selecting tasks in his or her job. This sense of choice is tied into employee empowerment. The employer provides autonomy to the employee when making decisions. A **sense of competence** is the feeling that occurs when an employee performs a challenging job well. The challenge level of the job relates to the competence level. This sense is related to job enrichment and job rotation. A **sense of meaningfulness** is the feeling an employee experiences when performing a task that contributes to organizational goals. For example, many healthcare employees experience a sense of meaningfulness because their tasks are directly related to patient welfare. Finally, a **sense of progress**, which is tied to a sense of meaningfulness, is the feeling that an employee's tasks are progressing forward and that the employee is not wasting time in performing tasks. In health care, an employee that is managing the chronic disease of a patient feels a sense of progress if the patient physically or mentally feels better.

In general, if employees feel they are being treated unfairly, their performance will suffer. It is important that an organization demonstrate both procedural and distributive justice. **Procedural justice** occurs when the process or procedures of allocating outcomes is perceived as fair or equitable. **Distributive justice** is the employees' perception of how rewards are allocated. **Interactional justice** focuses on how employees are actually treated by an organization when outcomes are distributed (Knicki & Kreitner, 2009). This is particularly important if an organization has to downsize and reduce the number of employees: If an employer sends an e-mail informing employees without notice or tells one employee personally and tells other employees via e-mail, the employer is not practicing interactional justice.

Motivational Strategies for Employee Performance

Thomas (2000) also developed four building blocks for his four types of intrinsic rewards. For his sense of choice, employers should (1) delegate authority to encourage employee decision making, (2) establish an organizational culture of worker trust, and (3) provide employees with adequate information to make decisions, and finally (4) employees should feel secure if they make honest mistakes as long as they do not compromise the safety of patients or other employees. This is important in healthcare organizations because much of the workload is often fulfilled by teams. Therefore, developing a culture of trust for each of the employees and teams can result in high team performance.

For a sense of competence, an employer should provide employee training to ensure an adequate level of knowledge for employees to perform their jobs. Supervisors should also provide positive feedback when an employee performs at a high level, recognizing his or her skills. Employees should also be challenged by establishing attainable goals to encourage a high level of performance. Health care is constantly changing with increased use of technology and changing regulations, therefore continuous training provided by the organization is needed. For example, the healthcare industry requires extensive safety measures for many employees' activities. There are traditional approaches to employee motivation for safety such as speakers, posters and signs, punitive action, and/or awards and incentives. They all have value, but, based on the theories described in the previous paragraphs, employees must value the motivation for promoting safety success. Regardless of the chosen approach, employees should be engaged in the safety improvement process. Asking for employee participation in developing and maintaining a safe work environment increases and encourages employees to achieve these goals because they participated in the process and attached a valence or value to the process (Krause, 2000).

To achieve a sense of meaningfulness, an employer establishes a motivating strategic vision that encourages employees to perform. Employees are given tasks that contribute to the organizational goal. A sense of progress should be supported by a collaborative organizational culture that celebrates milestones and employee accomplishments. A system measures employee performance. In 2009, the National Quality Forum contracted with the U.S. Department of Health and Human Services to establish performance measures for improving healthcare quality. These measures focus on patient conditions that account for more than 90% of Medicare costs (HHS Performance Measurement, 2011). Based on these measures, strategies will be developed to improve performance.

■ Training and Professional Development Programs

Training and professional development programs for employees are implemented to increase the knowledge of an employee. **Training programs** are typically developed to increase employee performance (Byars & Rue, 2006). Employees are trained to develop specific KSAs that are used in their jobs. Like training programs, **professional development programs** are targeted to employees, but the programs have broader knowledge goals, which can be applied to an employee's career goals. In addition to these types of training programs, other training programs are often implemented that are more behavior based. Such training programs include diversity in the workplace, business ethics, workplace safety, correction of performance issues, teamwork training, and cross-cultural training.

Organizational and Personnel Needs Assessment

Prior to implementation of any training initiatives, a **needs assessment** or evaluation is completed to determine types of training needed (Mathis & Jackson, 2006). The first component of the needs assessment is organizational analysis. The organization's corporate strategy must be assessed to determine the training needed. For example, if an organization is expanding its operations overseas or is increasing the number of foreign employees in its domestic operations, then cross-cultural and diversity training should be provided. If an organization must downsize, the remaining employees may need to be cross-trained in different jobs.

Another aspect of the **organizational needs assessment** is to determine what training infrastructure is in place. Some organizations have the ability to provide simulations and e-training rather than traditional class lectures. Some organizations offer in-house training, and others contract or outsource the training. These parameters must be assessed prior to development of a training structure.

Employee Analysis

The second component of the needs assessment for training is the assessment of individual employees, or **employee analysis**. The following questions should be answered: (1) Does an employee lack the skills or knowledge to perform his or her job well? (2) Does the employee need training in other areas such as diversity, safety, or cross-culture? Then, based on the answers to the first two questions, a list of employees is prepared.

Task Analysis

The third component of the needs assessment is **task analysis** (i.e., analysis of specific activities that are part of a job). Several tasks are part of a job position. Managers need to identify the skills and knowledge needed to perform a task well. The task analysis is used as the benchmark to compare with the employee assessment to determine what training is needed for the employee to complete the tasks well.

■ Training Versus Professional Development Programs

Training was identified earlier as a program that is specifically given to employees to improve their job performance by improving their KSAs. Professional development programs are more general and target employees' career goals, not just specifically the jobs they are currently performing (Noe, Hollenbeck, Gerhart & Wright, 2011). The knowledge gained in a professional development program may be used when an employee is promoted or if he or she is moved to another position. If your employer asks you to attend a professional development program, it may mean the employer believes that you have the qualifications and potential to be promoted, and the offer should be accepted.

■ Planning the Training and Professional Development Programs

The healthcare industry has varied environments that require different training programs; therefore goals are established for these training programs. For example, a hospital training program may have varied levels of training because of the different employees hired such as physicians, nurses, and technicians, whereas a physician's office training for employees would be less complex because the office is a smaller operation.

Participants must be identified for training programs. All new employees would require training; however, existing employees might also need training. A **readiness for training** determines whether an existing employee is interested in participating in the training and has the ability to learn (Dessler, 2012).

The healthcare organization must decide whether the training will be provided by the organization itself or outsourced to another company. Does the organization have the capabilities within to provide training?

Finally, the type of training methods must be identified. These decisions should be made based on employee input and surveys of other organizational programs. Evaluation of past training programs can be used to evaluate current programs.

Succession Planning

Organizations need to implement succession planning before they offer professional development programs. **Succession planning** consists of establishing a long-term plan for the replacement of important employees (Thompson, Strickland & Gamble, 2010). As stated earlier, professional development programs are offered to employees that have potential for promotion; therefore it is important to assess the strategic plan of the company to determine long-term labor needs and to assess potential labor shortages due to employee turnover, both voluntary and involuntary. Establishing a time frame for professional development programs will enable the organization to have employees at the ready to fill future vacated or new positions.

■ Training Methods

Once an employee is hired, his or her first training session is an **orientation**, which consists of an introduction to the organization and its policies and procedures (Mathis & Jackson, 2006). The length of the orientation program is dependent on the complexity of the organization. An orientation can be 1 day or 1 week. Orientation consists of an overview of the organization and the department of the new employee; HR issues such as employee benefits, policies, and procedures; and an introduction to the employee's job. Most employees are provided specific computer training. During an orientation, an employee will often receive an employee handbook, which the employee may sign for to indicate the receipt of the material. Orientation is an important introduction to the new employee's career at the organization. Anonymous evaluations of the orientation should be obtained to determine its effectiveness. Surveying existing employees about the orientation may also provide important feedback.

On-the-Job Training

On-the-job training is **informal training** that involves the new employee and colleagues who provide advice about the workplace and job. A new employee will observe an established employee while he or she performs the daily tasks. **Internships** and apprenticeships are types of on-the-job training. Internships are often established through relationships with academic institutions. Upper-level students in colleges or universities are assigned as interns in an organization. Depending on the length of the internship, students may receive credit for the internship or may receive a small stipend. Internships provide an opportunity for students to learn what it is like to work in a specific industry. In many academic programs, internships are required. Internships may lead to full-time employment.

Many medical students serve as interns at different healthcare facilities to assist with their career preference by providing on-the-job exposure (Byars & Rue, 2006). Many healthcare graduate and undergraduate students are required to perform internships as part of their degree requirement. As for medical internships, healthcare internships provide a glimpse into healthcare organizations. Some organizations hire individuals who have participated in internships because the organization already is familiar with the performance of the individual through his or her participation in the in-house internship program. An internship represents a wonderful opportunity for an individual to experience, on a short-term basis, different job aspects. It may help an individual to decide if the job or the career path is actually the correct one for him or her.

Apprenticeships are skilled trade programs such as carpentry and plumbing. The U.S. Department of Labor's Office of Apprenticeships, Registered Apprenticeship Model, has 40 programs that address labor shortages and increased demand for skilled workers. The model is a "learn while you earn" method that combines on-the-job training, instruction, and wages earned while on the job. Upon completion of the apprenticeship, the apprentice will earn a certificate that can be applied nationally. For example, a certified nursing assistant level 1 certificate requires 150 hours of training; level 2 requires 1000 hours, resulting in wage increase and an advanced certificate of training. Level 3 apprenticeships focus on hospice care, geriatrics, and dementia (U.S. Department of Labor, 2010).

Classroom Instruction and Computer-Based Training

Classroom instruction is a common method of providing information to employees. Traditionally, employees would attend classroom instruction in the organization's building. However, with the advent of computer technology, classroom instruction can be delivered electronically. Distance learning programs allow employees to train at different locations via video conferencing. Employees can take **webinars** (web-based classes) via an organization's distance learning programs. Many of these electronic offerings can be taken at the convenience of the employees outside usual work hours (Dessler, 2012). Participants may learn in interactive courses online, take exams, and participate in chat rooms. Computer-based training is less expensive and can be more easily customized to employees.

Audiovisual Training

Audiovisual training is another electronic offering that uses classroom material, but it is provided on CDs, DVDs, or as **podcasts**, which are downloaded lectures for iPods. There are many quality videos on YouTube that can be used for instruction. An advantage to offering portable electronic information is the ability of the participant to review the material for further clarification.

Simulations

A **simulation** is a training method that imitates real-life situations and enables employees to make decisions that would mirror real-life situations but without the risk. Simulations are very important in the healthcare industry because many decisions may be life threatening. Simulations allow employees to practice their decision making. In 2004, the Society for Simulation in Healthcare was established to support the increased use of simulation. Simulations that are offered online enable employees to create **avatars**, which are simulated people that the employees manipulate to reflect their knowledge while performing a task (About SSH, 2011).

Virtual Realty

Virtual reality (VR) is a computerized three-dimensional learning experience. It has become a key feature in training for minimally invasive surgical procedures in understaffed departments and for the completion of those procedures in actual operating rooms (Virtual Technologies Find Real Life Applications in Healthcare, 2011). The three-dimensional nature of VR allows the employee to view an object or environment from all sides and from its interior. A participant uses specialized equipment or can view an interactive environment three-dimensionally on a computer screen. A surgical unit of a hospital can use VR to practice surgery or to view the human body to assist with diagnosing a disease. A Healthcare IT report found that between 2006 and 2010, the U.S. market for health-related VR applications experienced a compound annual growth rate of more than 10%, reaching about $670 million in sales in 2010 (Market for Healthcare Virtual Reality Systems to Grow, 2011).

■ Types of Healthcare Training

Employees may participate in **experiential programs**, which mimic real-life situations in the training programs. **Case studies** are an example of experiential learning (Noe et al., 2011). Case studies are written narratives that provide facts about a real-life or fictitious situation in the healthcare industry. Questions are asked of the trainee about the narrative that focus on the trainee's behavior in the described situation. The goal of case studies is to develop critical thinking in students. Case studies enable the trainee to practice his or her response to a projected real-life situation in health care.

Diversity and Cultural Awareness Training

Because of continued labor shortages, healthcare organizations hire international employees. In addition to this trend, the labor laws that focus on antidiscrimination hiring have increased the hiring of more diverse employees at all management levels. Organizations such as the American Organization of Nurse Executives, American College of Healthcare Executives, and the Council on Graduate Medical Education have performed research on diversity issues in the healthcare industry that recognized the importance of diversity training. Organizations realize that different perspectives and backgrounds increase an organization's value to its customers (Salisbury & Byrd, 2006). This is certainly true in health care. Healthcare consumers are from diverse backgrounds and are more comfortable selecting a provider that has a similar background. **Diversity training** focuses on increasing awareness of individual differences. The goal is to make healthcare services **culturally competent,** which means behaviors, attitudes, and policies in an organization create an effective cross-cultural work environment (What Is Cultural Competency, 2011). The Office of Minority Health, U.S. Department of Health and Human Services, was created in 1985 to improve the health of minority populations through the development of health policies. Its position is that different cultures and languages will affect a healthcare consumer's and a healthcare provider's perception of the wellness system and that training must be performed to ensure differences are respected.

A diversity training program consists of three major components: legal, cultural, and sensitivity awareness (Mathis & Jackson, 2006). **Legal awareness training** is the most important component and provides training on legal discrimination. **Cultural awareness training** educates employees on the differences among nationalities and ethnicities. **Sensitivity awareness training** builds on cultural awareness training by focusing on the impact of actions by employees. Diversity training should be customized to the cultural and diversity needs of the organization and customer base. It must be supported by leadership, included in the organization's strategic plan, and implemented continually (Fried & Fottler, 2008).

Safety Training

The **Occupational Safety and Health Act** was passed in 1970 to ensure worker safety and to legislate that an organization has a general duty to provide a work environment free from hazards. **Job hazard analysis technique,** building on the job analysis, examines each job task, rating each task for any potential safety issue. Either the hazardous activity is changed or the employee is retrained if the employee was not performing the task safely. The **technic of operations review** analyzes job tasks that led to an accident. The circumstances of the workplace accident are reviewed and analyzed to determine which activity caused the accident. The employee will be retrained if necessary or the action will be eliminated (Dessler, 2012). Employees should be trained and evaluated regularly regarding safety procedures. In addition to training programs, incentive programs should reward employee safety practices to encourage safe behavior. In addition to employee safety training, safety information should be given to each employee to review any procedures.

It is difficult to ensure that safety practices are continued in an international setting. Many countries have different safety regulations. Organizations must develop a standardized policy for workplace safety, regardless of geographic location. Adoption of a standardized model ensures a safe work environment.

Business Ethics Training

Legal standards are the minimal standard of action established for individuals in a society. Ethical standards are considered to be one level above legal standards because individuals make a choice based on what is the "right thing to do" not what is required by law. There are many interpretations of the concept of ethics. Ethics has been interpreted as the moral foundation for standards of conduct (Taylor, 1975). The concept of **ethical standards** applies to actions that are hoped for and expected by individuals. Actions may be considered legal but not ethical. There are many definitions of ethics, but **ethics** is concerned with what are right and wrong choices as perceived by society and its individuals.

The concept of ethics is tightly woven throughout the healthcare industry. It has been dated back to Hippocrates, the father of medicine, who lived during the 4th century B.C., and evolved into the Hippocratic Oath, which is the foundation for the ethical guidelines for patient treatment by physicians. In 1847, the American Medical Association published a *Code of Medical Ethics* that provided guidelines for the physician–patient relationship, emphasizing the duty to treat a patient (Medical Ethics, 2011). To this day, physicians' actions have followed codes of ethics that demand the "duty to treat" (Wynia, 2007).

There is an impact on ethics in providing health care. Ethical dilemmas are often a conflict between personal and professional ethics. A **healthcare ethical dilemma** is a problem, situation, or opportunity that requires an individual, such as a healthcare provider, or an organization, such as a managed care practice, to choose an action that could be unethical (Niles, 2011).

Organizational ethics training can be delivered through classroom training, online training, or simulation training. An employee handbook may have a section on ethics training. Training should include informed consent, confidentiality, special populations, research ethics, ethics in public health, end-of-life decisions, genetic testing and profiling, and biomedical ethics and is reinforced throughout the employee's career with an organization.

Training to Correct Performance Problems

Every employee receives an appraisal of his or her job performance. Typically, an employee receives an annual review; however, new employees may have a probation period, which means they will be reviewed within 3 to 6 months of their initial hire. If an employee receives a favorable review, no training is needed to improve his or her performance. If the employee receives an unfavorable performance appraisal, training is needed to correct the problem. The problem may be the result of poor performance of a task or an attitude problem. Specific issues are identified to provide appropriate training to improve the employee's performance. Providing a plan of action to correct the employee's behavior gives the employee an opportunity to improve his or her performance.

Efficiency and Professional Development Training: Job Redesign

Job redesign is a professional development opportunity for an employee. It consists of job enlargement, job rotation, and job enrichment. Both job enlargement and job enrichment are common in health care. Job rotation is rarer in the healthcare industry because many jobs require a certification or license, so it would be more difficult to cross-train an employee unless he or she is willing to obtain the license or certification.

An employee may need additional training for the enlargement or increase of his or her responsibilities. In **job enlargement**, the employee expands his or her existing job tasks, depending on the needs of the organization and the strengths of the employee. In **job enrichment**, the employee receives an increase in responsibilities at a higher level. In any professional development training, it is a hint to the employee that the organization believes in his or her abilities and is providing the employee with the opportunity to expand his or her job capabilities.

Teamwork Training

The healthcare industry commonly performs teamwork. The care of a patient is provided by a team, not just the provider. According to Chinn (2010), quality teamwork performance contains the following characteristics: shared leadership, communication, and monitoring of all team performance. **Shared leadership** consists of all team members participating in the implementation of the decisions, rather than one team member making all of the decisions. This procedure is tied closely to the importance of team communications. Finally, team performance is monitored and evaluated to ensure that the best outcome was achieved. If the best outcome was not achieved, then a reevaluation of the team activity is performed.

■ Evaluation of Training Programs

Regardless of the goal of the training program, an evaluation component is required to assess if the program achieved its stated goal. Did the training positively alter the skills, knowledge, or abilities of an employee as it relates to his or her job? The purpose of a **transfer of training** is to evaluate any on-the-job use of the training material (Noe et al., 2011). In addition, any training programs can be evaluated by an online test or a simulation to assess the trainee's knowledge. A pretest of the trainee's KSAs and a posttest of the trainee's KSAs after the training can identify the impact of the training program.

■ Conclusion

Hughes (2003) and Trautman (2005) have developed tips for motivating employees that can be applied to healthcare organizations:

1. **Orientation:** Provide an in-depth orientation program for new employees.
2. **Incentives:** Providing incentives for quality performance will encourage the performance of other employees. This addresses any issues related to expectancy theory.

3. **Careful criticism:** Criticism is based solely on performance using standards for all employees. This addresses any issues of equity theory including procedural, distributive, and interactional justice.
4. **Routine performance of employee appraisals:** Employees need routine feedback to maintain, improve, or increase performance.
5. **Coaching and mentoring:** Instituting relationships with experienced employees provides a way to communicate organizational knowledge.
6. **Training and employee career development:** Providing opportunities to contribute to an employee's job performance and career encourages quality performance.
7. **Empowerment of employees:** Trusting employees to make decisions instills freedom for employees to continue to grow and enhance their performance.
8. **Management by objectives:** Asking for input from employees about their performance creates an atmosphere of empowerment and freedom to perform at a high level.
9. **Dedication of senior management:** Senior management must be dedicated to the organization, believe in the mission and vision of the organization, and act as role models for employees.
10. **Management transparency:** Senior management provides information on a continual basis to employees about the organizational operations. Employees have the opportunity to pursue any issues with senior management openly.

Motivation of healthcare employees can be achieved in different ways. Provision of both extrinsic and intrinsic rewards is appropriate. Employee training and development programs are motivational. There are several different motivational theories described in this chapter that can improve employee performance. In health care, high productivity is vital. If employees are not satisfied, their job performance will suffer. Nurses suffer from burnout because of high patient-to-nurse ratios. A high patient-to-nurse ratio also causes a lower quality of care because nurses do not have time to provide quality care, and if they are dissatisfied in general, the quality of work suffers. Employee burnout causes high employee turnover, which results in high organizational operating costs.

■ Vocabulary

Apprenticeships	Culturally competent
Audiovisual training	Distributive justice
Avatars	Diversity training
Case studies	Employee analysis
Cultural awareness training	Equity theory

Ethical standards
Ethics
Expectancy theory
Experiential programs
External rewards
Extrinsic rewards
Goal-setting theory
Healthcare ethical dilemma
Informal training
Interactional justice
Internal rewards
Internships
Intrinsic rewards
Job enlargement
Job enrichment
Job hazard analysis technique
Job redesign
Legal awareness training
Motivation
Needs assessment
Occupational Safety and Health Act
On-the-job training

Orientation
Podcasts
Procedural justice
Professional development programs
Readiness for training
Sense of choice
Sense of competence
Sense of meaningfulness
Sense of progress
Sensitivity awareness training
Shared leadership
Simulation
Succession planning
Task analysis
Technique of operations review
Training
Training programs
Transfer of training
Valence
Virtual reality
Webinars

■ References

About SSH (2011). Available at: http://www.ssih.org/SSIH/ssih/Home/AboutSSH/Default.aspx. Accessed February 13, 2011.

Aiken, L, Clarke, S., Sloane, D., Sochalski, J. & Silber, J. (2002). Hospital nurse staffing and patient mortality, nurse burnout and job dissatisfaction. *Journal of the American Medical Association*, 288(16):1993.

Buchbinder, S. & Shanks, N. (2007). *Introduction to Healthcare Management*. Sudbury, MA: Jones and Bartlett Publishers, pp. 23–34.

Byars, L. & Rue, L. (2006). *Human Resource Management* (8th ed.). New York, NY: McGraw-Hill/Irwin, pp. 371–383.

Chinn, D. (2010). Factors that promote effective teamwork in healthcare. Available at: http://www.ehow.com/list_6778245_factors-effective-teamwork-health-care.html. Accessed February 20, 2011.

Dessler, G. (2012). *Fundamentals of Human Resource Management*. Upper Saddle River, NJ: Prentice Hall, pp. 404–419.

Fried, B. & Fottler, M, (2008). *Human Resources in Health Care* (3rd ed.). Chicago, IL: Health Administration Press.

HHS Performance Measurement (2011). Available at: http://www.qualityforum.org/projects/ongoing/hhs/. Accessed March 6, 2011.

Hitt, M., Miller, C. & Colella, A. (2006). *Organizational Behavior: A Strategic Approach*. Hoboken, NJ: John Wiley & Sons, pp. 194–232.

Hughes, L. (2003). Motivating your employees. *WIB*, March/April:17.

Knicki, A. & Kreitner, R. (2009). *Organizational Behavior: Key Concepts, Skills & Practices*. New York, NY: McGraw-Hill/Irwin, pp. 174–187.

Krause, T. (2000). Motivating employees for safety success. *American Society of Safety Engineers*, March:22–25.

Lowe, G. (2002). High-quality healthcare workplaces: A vision and action plan. *Hospital Quarterly*, Summer:49–56.

Market for Healthcare Virtual Reality Systems to Grow (2011). Available at http://www.ihealthbeat.org/articles/2011/2/8/market-for-health-care-virtual-reality-systems-to-grow-report-says.aspx. Accessed January 9, 2012.

Mathis, R. & Jackson, J. (2006). *Human Resource Management* (11th ed.). Mason, OH: Thomson/South-Western, pp. 524–565.

Medical Ethics (2011). Available at: http://www.ama-assn.org/ama/pub/physician-resources/medical-ethics.html. Accessed December 15, 2011.

Niles, N. (2011). *Basics of the U.S. Health Care System*. Sudbury, MA: Jones & Bartlett Learning: 250–255.

Noe, R., Hollenbeck, J., Gerhart B. & Wright, P. (2011). *Fundamentals of Human Resource Management* (3rd ed.). New York, NY: McGraw-Hill/Irwin, pp. 29–30.

Salisbury, J. & Byrd, S. (2006). Why diversity matters in health care. *CSA Bulletin*, Spring:90–93.

Taylor, P. (1975). *Principles of Ethics: An Introduction*. Encino, CA: Dickson Publishing Co.

Thomas, K. (2000). Intrinsic motivation and how it works. *Training*, October:130–135. Available at: http://www.evaluationengineering.com/index.php/solutions/management-and-career/my-top-10-practices-for-leading-and-motivating-a-workforce.html. Accessed March 6, 2011.

Thompson, A., Strickland, A. & Gamble, J. (2010). *Crafting & Executing Strategy: The Quest for Competitive Advantage*. Boston, MA: McGraw-Hill/Irwin, pp. 1–15.

Trautman, J. (2005). My top 10 practices for leading and motivating a workforce. Available at: http://www.highbeam.com/doc/1G1-135082130.html. Accessed December 13, 2011

U.S. Department of Labor (2010). Using registered apprenticeships to build and fill healthcare career paths. Available at: http://www.doleta.gov/oa/pdf/Apprenticeship_Build_HealthCare_Paths.pdf. Accessed February 13, 2011.

Virtual Technologies Find Real Life Applications in Healthcare (2011). Available at: http://www.kaloramainformation.com/about/release.asp?id=1873. Accessed February 20, 2011.

What Is Cultural Competency? (2011). Available at: http://minorityhealth.hhs.gov/templates/browse.aspx.?lvl=2&lv1ID=11. Accessed February 20, 2011.

Wynia, M. (2007). Ethics and public health emergencies. Encouraging responsibility. *The Amercian Journal of Bioethics*, 7, 1–4.

STUDENT WORKBOOK ACTIVITY 7.1

Complete the following case scenarios based on the information provided in this chapter. Your responses must be *in our own words*.

Real-Life Applications: Case Scenario 1

As the manager of a department of radiology, you just hired five new radiologists. You need to develop an initial training plan for them.

Activity

Define and describe the first training program the new employees should receive and the components of this type of training.

Responses

_____

_____

_____

_____

_____

Real-Life Applications: Case Scenario 2

You are a newly hired healthcare administrator at a local hospital. The hospital has experienced recent high turnover in the nursing sector. Exit strategies with the employees indicate they felt they were unfairly treated, there was no feedback from senior management regarding employee performance, and they had no participation in the performance appraisal process.

Activity

Develop a motivational strategy to reduce turnover in the nursing sector.

_____

_____

_____

_____

Real-Life Applications: Case Scenario 3

Your supervisor just read about the importance of intrinsic motivation of employees and about Thomas's four-prong model of motivation. He has asked you to develop a plan utilizing Thomas's approach that can be used to motivate employees.

Activity

Explain the difference between intrinsic and extrinsic rewards. Explain the Thomas model and provide four different types of activities for this type of organization.

Responses

_____

_____

_____

_____

Real-Life Applications: Case Scenario 4

A new laboratory will be opening in 6 months that is owned by the local hospital. The hospital needs to train 25 laboratory technicians. They have already received orientation from the hospital, but senior management feels they need additional training. As the manager, you have been asked to develop a safety-training program for these new employees.

Activity

Identify the important components of the safety program for these employees. Include any analysis techniques that would be needed in the safety program. Discuss any legal requirements for this type of program.

Responses

_____

_____

_____

_____

_____

STUDENT WORKBOOK ACTIVITY 7.2

In Your Own Words

Please describe these core concepts in your own words.

Equity theory:

_____

_____

_____

_____

Intrinsic rewards:

_____

_____

_____

_____

Transfer of training:

_____

_____

_____

_____

Readiness for training:

_____

_____

_____

_____

Succession planning:

_____

_____

_____

_____

Expectancy theory:

_____

_____

_____

_____

Valence:

_____

_____

_____

_____

Interactional justice:

_____

_____

_____

_____

STUDENT WORKBOOK ACTIVITY 7.3

Internet Exercises

Write your answers in the spaces provided.

- Visit each of the websites that are listed in the text that follows.
- Name the organization.
- Locate its mission statement on its website. If the organization does not have a mission statement, describe its purpose.
- Provide a brief overview of the activities of the organization.
- Apply this organization to the chapter information.

Websites
www.intrahealth.org
Organization name:

_____

Mission statement:

_____

_____

_____

Overview of activities:

_____

_____

_____

Application to chapter information:

_____

_____

_____

http://www.whpa.org
Organization name:

_____

Mission statement:

_____

_____

_____

Overview of activities:

_____

_____

_____

Application to chapter information:

_____

_____

_____

http://www.medscape.com

Organization name:

_____

Mission statement:

_____

_____

_____

Overview of activities:

_____

_____

_____

Application to chapter information:

_____

_____

_____

http://www.hrhresourcecenter.org/
Organization name:

_____

Mission statement:

_____

_____

_____

Overview of activities:

_____

_____

_____

Application to chapter information:

_____

_____

_____

http://curinghealthcare.blogspot.com
Organization name:

_____

Mission statement:

_____

_____

_____

Overview of activities:

_____

_____

_____

Application to chapter information:

_____

_____

_____

http://www.healthleadersmedia.com

Organization name:

_____

Mission statement:

_____

_____

_____

Overview of activities:

_____

_____

_____

Application to chapter information:

_____

_____

_____

STUDENT ACTIVITY 7.4: DISCUSSION BOARDS FOR ONLINE, HYBRID, AND TRADITIONAL ONGROUND CLASSES

Discussion Board Guidelines

The discussion board is used in online and web-enhanced courses in place of classroom lectures and discussion. The board can be an enhancement to traditional classes. The discussion board is the way in which the students "link together" as a class. The following are guidelines to help focus on the discussion topic and to define the roles and responsibilities of the discussion coordinator and other members of the class. The educator will be the discussion moderator for this course.

1. The educator will post the discussion topic and directions for the upcoming week. These postings should all be responses to the original topic or responses to other students' responses. When people respond to what someone else has posted, they should start the posting with the person's name so it is clear which message they are responding to. **A response such as "Yes" or "I agree" does not count for credit. Your responses must be in your own words. You cannot copy and paste from the text.**

2. Postings (especially responses) should include enough information so the message is clear but should not be so long that it becomes difficult to follow. Remember, this is like talking to someone in a classroom setting. The postings should reflect the content of the textbook or other assignments. If you retrieve information from the Internet, the hyperlink must be cited.

3. Students should check the discussion daily to see if new information has been posted that requires their attention and response.

Good discussion will often include different points of view. Students should feel free to disagree or "challenge" others to support their positions or ideas. All discussions must be handled in a respectful manner. The following are discussion boards for this chapter.

Discussion Boards

1. In your own words, define motivation. Discuss three ways managers can motivate employees.
2. What is the difference between training and professional development? Describe your training and professional development experiences that were motivating or not motivating to you.
3. Do you think the healthcare industry is diverse? Describe how you would develop a cross-cultural training program for employees who work in a diverse environment.
4. Can workers be trained in ethics? How? Defend your answer.

Employee Relations

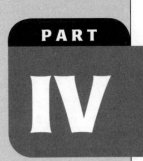

Labor Unions and Health Care

The student will be able to:

- Discuss the history of U.S. labor unions.
- Analyze the impact of labor unions on health care.
- List the steps in forming a union.
- Evaluate the impact of unions on nurses.
- Assess the impact of unions on physicians.
- Describe the impact of strikes on patient care.

DID YOU KNOW THAT?

- The National Nurses United union, called the "super union," is the largest nurses union and professional organization of U.S. nurses.
- Hospitals are the primary employers of nurses.
- In some instances, managed care models reduced physician income by 40%.
- Recent statistics indicate that there are nearly 3 million employed nurses in the United States.
- U.S. union membership has declined except in the healthcare industry.

■ Introduction

Because of the economic revolution in the United States, President William Howard Taft established the U.S. Department of Labor in 1913. Its mission was and is to promote the welfare of working people and the decency of their working conditions. By the end of World War I, the U.S. Department of Labor had established policies to ensure fair wages and decent working conditions so that human resources, employees, were treated fairly (Grossman, 1973). Early **labor union** organizations were established from the late 1700s to early 1800s because employees believed that management was not treating them fairly with respect to wages and hours. Early membership labor organizations represented different types of skilled employees, such as printers or carpenters, to ensure the fair treatment of the employees by management. Labor unions focused on job security, fair wages, and shorter working hours. Union membership reached its peak in the 1950s, but has declined over the past 20 years in many industries. Labor unions can be regarded as the predecessors of human resources departments (Byars & Rue, 2006). The goal of both is the equitable treatment of employees by management.

Despite the decrease in union membership, healthcare unions are increasing in strength, particularly in the nursing sector. In 2007, the Service Employees International Union (SEIU) created a national healthcare union, which is the largest healthcare union nationally. SEIU Healthcare represents hospital, nursing, long-term care, and many outpatient facility workers, and SEIU-affiliated unions represent physicians also. In 2010, the California Nurses Association and the United American Nurses merged and the Massachusetts Nurses Association created National Nurses United, the largest nurses union in the United States, representing 150,000 members (Malvey, 2010). This chapter will describe the history of U.S. union development, how unions are formed, legislation that affects unions, and the impact of unions on the healthcare industry.

■ History of U.S. Unions

Unions are membership labor organizations formed to protect their members' employee rights. Their main goal is to ensure that management treats its employees fairly. Although there were U.S. workers who organized them against unfair management practices in the 1700–1800s, it was not until 1935 that the **National Labor Relations Act** (Wagner Act) was passed to protect the right of workers to form unions. It also defined unfair labor practices and established the National Labor Relations Board (NLRB), which is responsible for National Labor Relations Act (NLRA) regulatory oversight. This is the only federal legislation that protects labor relations by allowing employees to form unions. Because of this legislation, union membership nearly tripled (Gentry, 2008). Section 7 of the act also allows **collective bargaining**, which is a labor relations term that refers to union negotiation with management for employment parameters such as wages and other benefits for the employees. The NLRB also ensures that union elections are fair. Between the 1950s and 1970s, union membership represented more than 25% of the U.S. workforce. The NLRA was amended in 1947 and 1959 by the Taft–Hartley Act and the Landrum–Griffin Act, respectively. Section 14b of the **Taft–Hartley Act** permitted states to pass right-to-work laws that supported the freedom of employees to choose whether to join a union or not. This act also permitted the president of the United States to declare that strikes or employee work stoppages as a means of protesting employee conditions could affect the national economy, thereby forcing union members to return to work without resolving their issues. This act exempted not-for-profit hospitals from NLRA coverage and was amended in 1974 (the Healthcare Amendments) to include private, not-for-profit hospitals and nursing homes. The act also instituted stricter rules regarding work stoppages to increase patient care protection, and it required 10-day strike and picket notices to employers to ensure that healthcare institutions would have ample notice of such activity. If employees do not respect the 10-day notice, they lose their status as employees. The **Landrum–Griffin Act** protected the rights of union members with respect to union meeting participation and review of union financial records. It also required unions to establish bylaws (Mathis & Jackson, 2006).

In 1989, an NLRB ruling declared eight units eligible for collective bargaining in acute-care hospitals: registered nurses; physicians; all other professionals such as social workers, physician therapists, and pharmacists; technical employees; clerical employees; skilled maintenance employees; all other nonprofessional employees; and security guards (Stickler & Gournis, 2010).

As the U.S. economy focused less on manufacturing and evolved into a service economy during the 1980s and 1990s, union membership declined. However, service industries such as health care are being targeted by union organizers because these industries are a large untapped source of potential union membership. In 2009, union membership represented 12% of all U.S. workers, which is a decrease from 24% in 1979. However, union membership in the healthcare industry is increasing slightly. In 2000, 12.9% of healthcare workers were unionized. In 2009, the percentage increased to 13.6%, or 1 million workers. Unions are hoping to increase their membership in the healthcare industry as the recession creates tension between workers and management via cost-cutting measures. Notably, the major reason unions are formed is that employees are dissatisfied with wages. Typically, a unionized worker earns more than 25% to 30% of the wage of a non-union worker, but in the healthcare industry, a typical unionized worker only earns more than 12% of the wage of a non-union employee (Elliott, 2010).

■ How Unions Organize

Unions assess organizations to determine if a union will be successful in the organization. Dissatisfied employees are a target for union organizers. Unions can be formed in two ways. A union can launch a campaign to convince employees that if they form a union, it will help them improve their working conditions. Internally, dissatisfied employees may also decide to form a union because they believe that employees are unhappy with management. Usually, wages and benefits are the cause of union formation.

A union campaign is an organized effort to persuade employees to form a union. A campaign may consist of printed and electronic media, individual contacts, and/or special meetings. The sole purpose of these efforts is for the employees to sign **union authorization cards** that designate the union as the representative of the employees to negotiate employee benefits. At least 30% of the employees must sign an authorization card in order to hold an election to vote on union formation. Prior to the election, a bargaining unit must be designated. A **bargaining unit** is recognized by the employer as an appropriate group of employees who work in the same industry classification, have similar working conditions and wages, and have similar geographic location and supervisors. The bargaining unit is an organizational formation used for collective bargaining in labor negotiations (Mondy, 2012).

If at least 30% of the employees sign cards, then the next step is to hold an election by secret ballot. If more than 50% of the workers sign authorization cards, the union may ask management to recognize the union without an election. Both the NLRA and its amendments place restrictions on both sides with respect to organizing activities. Managers and unions may discuss wages, may exchange their points of view regarding unions, and may provide negative materials. Management can deny union distribution of materials at the workplace. Neither the union nor management can bribe the employees to vote for or against the union, threaten employees, ask the employees how they will be voting, or give campaign speeches 24 hours prior to the election. If an election is held, the union must receive a majority of votes to move forward. Once it is determined the election was fair, the NLRB certifies the election, and the union will represent its members in labor negotiations through the collective bargaining process (Mathis & Jackson, 2006).

■ Negotiating with Unions

Once a union has been established in an organization, it now has the right to negotiate on behalf of the member employees. The NLRA defines collective bargaining as an "obligation of the employer and union to meet and negotiate in good faith regarding conditions of employment and to execute a written agreement that is reached in good faith by both parties" (National Labor Relations Act, Section 8d, 2010).

Mandatory negotiation issues focus on wages, management and union rights, job security, and benefits including vacation, sick leave, and health insurance. When an agreement is reached by both parties, a written agreement is implemented. The key to effective collective bargaining is that both parties negotiate in good faith, meaning they agree to listen to each other with an open mind in order to reach a final agreement (Malvey, 2010). If both sides agree, a written agreement will be implemented that outlines all of the agreed-upon employment issues including disciplinary actions by management and grievance issues by employees. This agreement is clearly articulated to both sides so management and the employees understand how they must act in the workplace.

When Collective Bargaining Fails

If the collective bargaining process does not result in an agreement, the company ultimately does not want to pursue legal action or deal with an employee strike because of the cost and the damage to the reputation of the company. If an agreement cannot be reached, other avenues to reach agreement are pursued such as mediation or arbitration, which are alternative dispute resolution measures. **Alternative dispute resolution** represents methods other than the court system that are used to resolve labor issues. **Mediation** is an informal process and is widely used. A third party tries to negotiate an agreement between the two parties. The suggestion by the mediator is not binding, which means both parties do not have to abide by the ruling. **Arbitration** is a formal process that negotiates an agreement that is binding, which means it has to be respected by both parties. If the employees are truly dissatisfied, they may not opt for these processes and instead decide to strike. A **strike** is a work stoppage by the employees until a satisfactory agreement is met (Mathis & Jackson, 2006). It is unusual now for employees to strike. Both parties attempt to resolve issues via alternative dispute resolution measures.

■ Federal Mediation and Conciliation Service

Workers have been striking for centuries as a way of protesting unfair working conditions. In 1838, President Martin Van Buren settled a strike by shipyard workers, which was the first time the government mediated a labor settlement in the United States. In 1918, the **U.S. Department of Labor** created the U.S. Conciliation Service followed by the establishment of the National Mediation Board because of the Railway Labor Act, which allowed railroad unions to organize. The Federal Mediation and Conciliation Service (FMCS) was established in 1947 as part of the Taft–Hartley Act. The purpose of the FMCS is to minimize the effects of labor–management disputes on business operations. Since its establishment, the FMCS has been instrumental in resolving labor–management disputes through mediation and **conciliation** services. The NLRA requires 60 days' notice by the employers or employee representatives that a Collective Bargaining Agreement (CBA) is being modified or terminated. The FMCS is also notified in case its services are needed (Federal Mediation and Conciliation Services, 2010).

■ Individual Grievance Process

If an employee believes that management is not abiding by the collective bargaining agreement, the individual may grieve the issue. The **grievance procedure** is at the core of the CBA, of which the first step is for the employee to present the grievance to the immediate supervisor. If the supervisor is the issue, the employee will grieve at a higher level of management. The employee must present the grievance in writing, which is reviewed at each management level until it is resolved. Once the grievance is resolved, the review process stops. If the grievance cannot be resolved internally, a mediator or arbitrator will be introduced as discussed earlier (Byars & Rue, 2006).

■ History of Unions and the Healthcare Industry

Over the past several decades, legislation has focused on collective bargaining inclusion of different healthcare employee classifications. What is becoming more important in the collective bargaining agreements is the eligibility of certain management employees. Many healthcare organizations' goals are organized by team structures. Their organizational structures have become flatter with fewer levels of management concentration at higher levels of the organization, which creates confusion as to who is eligible and who is ineligible for union representation. Many employees who did not have a management role now have managerial responsibilities. Another issue is that eligibility of union membership is for employees only. Many healthcare employees may be independent contractors including nurses and physicians, which precludes them from union membership. These management trends must be clarified for unionization of certain healthcare employees (Sanders & McCutcheon, 2010).

There are two court cases that affect the supervisory status issues of nurses: Kentucky River Community Care, Inc. (*NLRB vs. Kentucky River Community Care, Inc.*, 532 U.S. 706 [2001]), and the Oakwood Healthcare, Inc. (*NLRB vs. Oakwood Healthcare Inc.*, 348, No. 37 [Sept. 29, 2006]). In 2001, with the U.S. Supreme Court decision *NLRB vs. Kentucky River Community Care, Inc.*, the Supreme Court opined that the NLRB was not clear in its definition of supervisory status of an employee and required the NLRB to develop a new test to determine supervisory status of nurses. The revised definition developed by NLRB included the concept of "**independent judgment**" as an activity of supervisors, which means that nurses who were considered supervisors must routinely direct other nurses. However, a nurse can avoid the supervisor status if the independent judgment is the result of specific regulations or employee orders from the nurse's supervisor. Using their revised definition of supervisory status, in the 2006 Oakwood Healthcare, Inc., case, the NLRB ruled that permanent charge nurses employed by the Oakwood Heritage Hospital were considered supervisors if they assigned and directed other nurses on a routine basis, which may result in their exclusion from the bargaining unit. However, the NLRB determined that if nurses were supervising other nurses on a part-time basis, they were eligible for union membership (Malvey, 2010). These two cases will continue the debate of whether certain nurses are considered management and whether they are excluded from union membership.

■ Nurses and Unions

Nearly 3 million nurses are employed in the United States. They are employed predominantly by hospitals. By 2016, there will be a need for 500,000 more nurses. There continues to be a nursing shortage in the United States. With labor shortages, nursing salaries have risen. The main labor issue with nurses is the working conditions. Healthcare organizations have experienced financial problems because of the recession. More nonpaying patients are using hospital services, which increases the bad debt and charity expenses of hospitals. As a result of fewer paying patients, there has been downsizing in organizations, which has resulted in increased patient loads for nurses. Nurses originally focused on legislation to enact nurse–patient ratios, but the powerful hospital lobbyists restricted that avenue, so nurses have used unions to negotiate nurse–patient ratios (Carlson, 2010). There are four dominant unions that represent nurses nationally: SEIU, California Nurses Association (CNA), United American Nurses (UAN), and American Nurses Association (ANA) (Benson, 2009). The SEIU has organized hospitals so that nurses and ancillary staff are represented together.

American Nurses Association (ANA)

The ANA was formed in 1911 as a non-union nurses association, but by the 1940s it started to unionize its members. By 2000, it established collective bargaining divisions that were joined as the UAN, which was controlled by the ANA. The UAN joined forces with the American Federation of Labor-Congress of Industrial Organizations (AFL-CIO) with the ANA as the administrator and financier of the UAN. In 2003, the UAN became independent of the ANA while maintaining a relationship with the ANA. By 2007, the UAN's membership was 108,000. The ANA denounced the UAN and terminated their relationship in 2008 (Benson, 2009). The ANA continues to be a powerful representative of nurses. ANANurseSpace is a social network for ANA members. The ANA also has a relationship with the Center for American Nurses, an advocacy organization (About ANA, 2010).

California Nurses Association/National Nurses Organizing Committee to National Nurses United

The CNA also started as a membership organization for nurses in management. In 1993, staff nurses took it over from management nurses and developed it into a labor organization with a collective bargaining focus. In 2006, it became affiliated with the AFL-CIO. It has evolved from representing California nurses to the National Nurses Organizing Committee (NNOC) with 86,000 members in hospitals, home clinics, and home health agencies. Membership has grown 400% over the past 15 years (About the California Nurses Association/National Nurses Organizing Committee, 2010). In 2009, it became a founding member of National Nurses United (NNU), the largest nurses union, representing 155,000 registered nurses. It competes with SEIU for membership.

Service Employees International Union

The SEIU is the fastest growing union in the United States with nearly 2 million members. It focuses on long-term care, hospital systems, and nurse alliances. The SEIU's original name was Building Service Employees International Union, which had a focus on service in residential and commercial buildings. When the union opened its membership to the service industry, the union included healthcare employees. The SEIU Nurse Alliance represents 85,000 registered nurses in 21 states, but there appears to be discontent among its members. SEIU fears that the CNA can recruit unhappy members from the organization. The CNA is targeting states such as Texas, Nevada, and Ohio where SEIU nurses are unhappy with their representation. In 2005, the SEIU ended its relationship with the AFL-CIO, and in 2007, it established one of its sectors, SEIU Healthcare. SEIU negotiated a large labor contract with a private for-profit hospital chain in Florida. In 2010, the SEIU established a Nurse Alliance Quality Committees Program that focuses on health and safety, workplace quality, health information technology, policy, and training and education (2010 Nurse Alliance Quality Committees Program, 2010).

National Nurses United

In 2009, **National Nurses United** was established as the largest nurses union and professional organization of U.S. nurses. This "super union" was formed by three organizations: **United American Nurses, Massachusetts Nurses Association**, and **California Nurses Association/National Nurses Organizing Committee**. Its focus, like the focus of other unions, is on working conditions. Nurses continue to believe that they are not allowed adequate time to properly provide quality care to their patients (Who We Are, NNU, 2010).

■ Physicians Unions

As discussed earlier, employees who are independent contractors and employees who are considered supervisors are not eligible to participate in collective bargaining. For example, during the 1990s when managed care organizations (MCOs) became a tool to provide healthcare services, many physicians contracted with several MCOs that did not allow the physicians to collectively bargain because the physicians were independent contractors. Many physicians also managed their own practices, which also placed them in a supervisor capacity. Therefore, there were few physicians that were eligible to form unions. In addition, there existed unionization issues with respect to residents and interns (house staff). However, in a 1999 decision, the NLRB ruled that residents and interns were employees and therefore could unionize. This landmark decision contradicted decades of discussion regarding these individuals (Nijm & Liang, 2001). The physician membership organization and powerful lobbyist for its members, the American Medical Association (AMA), was historically against unions because the organization believed it would be detrimental to the quality of patient care. The physician has the responsibility to treat patients regardless of ability to pay. What would happen if the physicians went on a strike because they were unhappy with their working conditions or wages? However, the advent of managed care bothered the AMA, and in 1999 it created the **Physicians for Responsible Negotiations** (PRN). According to estimates, in many instances managed care reduced physician income by more than 40% even though average physician income was very high (Farmer & Douglas, 2010). Despite the impact of managed care, the PRN, with few members, was not successful. The AMA eventually severed its ties with the group in 2004. The PRN, however, joined the SEIU with two other physicians unions, **Doctors Council** and the **National Doctors Alliance**. These three unions represent approximately 20,000 physician members.

Committee of Interns and Residents, National Doctors Alliance, and Doctors Council

The **Committee of Interns and Residents** is part of the National Doctors Alliance (NDA). Doctors who are employees in a nonsupervisory capacity in a facility, hospital, university, medical center, or in private practice can join the NDA. Formed in 1973, the Doctors Council represents doctors employed in New York City. It is the sister organization of the Committee of Interns and Residents, founded in 1957 by New York City interns and residents, which is the largest house staff union in the country, representing 13,000 residents in several states. In 1958, it negotiated the first collective bargaining agreement for residents and interns. In 1975, it negotiated the first contractual agreements for on-call scheduling for residents and interns. In the 1990s, it negotiated set hours for house staff in New York State and in other states. These time limitations have been instrumental in establishing model programs throughout the United States. It is obvious that both the nurses and physicians unions have increased their strength by their affiliation with SEIU Healthcare. The adage "strength in numbers" certainly applies to the strategies of forming larger organizations (About CIR, 2010).

■ Allied Health Professionals Unions

Like the nurses and physicians unions, the unions that represent allied health professionals have joined forces, although efforts are primarily state-based with 15 unions. The Health Professionals and Allied Employees is the largest union of nurses and allied health employees in New Jersey, representing 12,000 members. In 1978, it became affiliated with AFT Healthcare, which is a healthcare division of the American

Federation of Teachers (AFT). The union membership includes nurses and medical researchers, dieticians, physicians, psychologists, X-ray technicians, and other healthcare professionals from 17 states. Members work in hospitals, nursing homes, schools, laboratories, blood banks, clinics, and home health agencies (About AFT Healthcare, 2010).

■ Conclusion

Regardless of the industry, unions are formed because employees are dissatisfied with their jobs. Either the wages are too low or the working conditions are poor. As healthcare expenditures continue to increase, healthcare reform will continue to focus on cost reduction. Managed care models targeted labor costs, which resulted in physicians and nurses becoming disgruntled because they were worried about quality of patient care (Schraeder & Friedman, 2002). Nurses formed unions because they were less concerned with wages than with quality working conditions to ensure patient care. Residents and interns were also concerned with working conditions because of the traditional long hours they endure while training. Establishing a union resulted in limited working hours for them. Allied health professional unions have been established to ensure that fair wages are being applied in their industry. It has been difficult for physicians unions to become more powerful because so many physicians are self-employed and are excluded from union membership. There are also exceptional health systems such as the Cleveland Clinic, which is excellent to its physician employees (Romano, 2001). With the advent of healthcare reform legislation and the reduction of reimbursement for physician services to Medicare and Medicaid patients, there may be more of a reason to organize. Over the past 5 years, unions won 70% of healthcare organizing efforts, with New York, California, and Illinois representing nearly 50% of the total elections (By the Numbers, 2009). In 2009, there were 11 strikes, which affected 2,600 workers, or 238 workers per strike, which is fairly low. In 2010, there were seven strikes involving 14,000 workers, or 2,000 workers per strike (Commis, 2010).

Regardless of goals, union formation in the healthcare industry is characterized by mergers of several unions to increase their voice in dealing with employers. Large unions such as the AFT and SEIU have established separate legal entities that represent healthcare issues. Although union membership has declined in the United States over the past decades, union membership in the healthcare industry has increased.

Particularly in the healthcare industry, it is important that employees are satisfied with their jobs and strive to perform at above-average levels. Dissatisfied employees may result in poor performance. Nurses are dissatisfied with their working conditions. These employees provide direct services to patients. The Institute of Medicine's research indicates that more than 80,000 to 100,000 errors occur each year leading to patient death as a result of improper treatment (Emanuel, 2008). The Agency for Healthcare Research and Quality recently supported that an increase in nurse staffing would improve patient safety and reduce negative patient care (Carlson, 2010). Therefore, from a management perspective, it is important that quality employees be retained. The following are suggestions for management to satisfy its unionized and non-union employees:

1. **Procedural justice:** It is important that employees perceive that they are being treated fairly and that methods to determine outcomes are standardized (Hitt, Miller & Colella, 2006). Job analyses, job descriptions, job specifications, job recruitment, and performance appraisals must be implemented objectively to ensure that employees believe they are being treated fairly with the outcomes of these procedures. Written standard operating procedures for each of these tasks must be developed to ensure there is objectivity for each of these categories.
2. **Employee training and development:** Employees must be trained for their positions to ensure they perform effectively. In addition to job performance, management must also be trained in the organization's policies in order to manage its employees effectively.
3. **Performance appraisals:** If an employee believes he or she is not being fairly evaluated on job performance, he or she may file a grievance or complain to senior management. Applying procedures fairly to all employees creates a culture of justice and avoids conflict.

Strikes can have a devastating impact on a healthcare organization, particularly when nurses go on strike, because any work stoppage could have a dramatic effect on quality of patient care. In a recent hospital study in New York, Gruber and Kleiner (2010) indicate that during the period 1984–2004, nurses' strikes led to a 19.4% increase of in-house mortality and a 6.5% increase in readmissions. Management should have a plan in place as described earlier that recognizes that employees are assets not just costs and, particularly in the healthcare industry, should be rewarded for quality performance.

■ Vocabulary

Alternative dispute resolution
Arbitration
Bargaining unit
California Nurses Association/
   National Nurses Organizing
   Committee
Collective bargaining
Committee of Interns and Residents
Conciliation
Doctors Council

Employee training and development
Grievance procedure
Independent judgment
Labor unions
Landrum–Griffin Act
Massachusetts Nurses Association
Mediation
National Doctors Alliance
National Labor Relations Act
National Nurses United

Performance appraisals
Physicians for Responsible
  Negotiations
Procedural justice
Strike

Taft–Hartley Act
Union authorization cards
Unions
United American Nurses
U.S. Department of Labor

■ References

About AFT Healthcare (2010). Available at: http://www.aft.org/yourwork.healthcare/about.cfm. Accessed November 14, 2010.

About ANA (2010). Available at: http://www.nursingworld.org/FunctionalMenuCategories/About ANA .aspx. Accessed November 14, 2010.

About CIR (2010). Available at: http://www.cirseiu.org/about/Default.aspx. Accessed November 10, 2010.

About the California Nurses Association/National Nurses Organizing Committee (2010). Available at: http://www.calnurses.org/about-us. Accessed November 7, 2010.

Benson, H. (2009). Who will organize 2.5 million nurses in the U.S.? *The Journal of Labor and Society*, 12:131–141.

Byars, L. & Rue, L. (2006). *Human Resource Management* (8th ed.). New York, NY: McGraw-Hill/ Irwin, pp 369–383.

By the Numbers (2009). *Modern Healthcare*, 36(44):9.

Carlson, J. (2010). Rallying for ratios. *WorkingUSA*, 40(24):8–9.

Commis, J. (2010). Healthcare unions post strong gains. Available at: http://www.healthldersmedia.com/ print/HR-257825/Healthcare-Unions-Post-Strong-Gains. Accessed November 20, 2010.

Elliott, V. (2010). Unions for healthcare workers are growing. Available at: http://www.ama-assn.org/ amednews/2010/02/22/bisb0222.htm. Accessed November 14, 2010.

Emanuel, E. (2008). *Health Care Guaranteed*. New York, NY: Public Affairs.

Farmer, G. & Douglas, J. (2010). Physician unionization: A primer and prescription. Available at: http:// www.floridabar.org/divcom/jn/jnjournal101.nsf. Accessed November 14, 2010.

Federal Mediation and Conciliation Services (2010). Who we are. Available at: http://www.fmcs.gov/ internet/itemDetail.asp?categoryID=21&itemID=15810. Accessed November 20, 2010.

Gentry, W. (2008). Health safety and preparedness. In Fried, B. & Fottler, M., eds. *Human Resources in Healthcare*. Chicago, IL: Health Administration Press, pp. 347–391.

Grossman, J. (1973). The origins of the U.S. Department of Labor. Available at: http://www.dol.gov/ oasam/programs/history/dolorigabridge.htm. Accessed December 20, 2011.

Gruber, J. & Kleiner, S. (2010). Do strikes kill? Evidence from New York State. Available at: http://www .nber.org/papers/w15855. Accessed November 20, 2010.

Hitt, M., Miller, C. & Colella, A. (2006). *Organizational Behavior: A Strategic Approach*. Hoboken, NJ: Wiley, pp. 200–220.

Malvey, D. (2010). Unionization in healthcare: Background and trends. *Journal of Healthcare Management*, 55(3):154–157.

Mathis, R. & Jackson, J. (2006). *Human Resource Management* (11th ed.). Mason, OH: Thomson/ South-Western, pp. 521–551.

Mondy, R. (2012). Human Resource Management. Upper Saddle River, NH: Prentice Hall, pp. 330–335.

National Labor Relations Act, Section 8(d) (2010). Available at: http://www.nlrb.gov/about_us/overview/national_labor_relations_act.aspx. Accessed November 20, 2010.

Nijm, L. & Liang, B. (2001). Physician unionization: White coats with blue collars. *Hospital Physician*, May:71–74.

Romano, M. (2001). No bargaining. *Modern Healthcare*, 31(22):12–14.

Sanders, L. & McCutcheon, A. (2010). Unions in the healthcare industry. *Labor Law Journal*, Fall: 142–151.

Schraeder, M. & Friedman, L. (2002). Collective bargaining in the nursing profession: Salient issues and recent developments in healthcare reform. *Hospital Topics*, 80(3):21–24.

Stickler, K. & Gournis, S. (2010). Special Considerations in the Health Care Industry. Available at: http://www.drinkerbiddle.com/files/Publication/6d5fd9ec-e610-4de7-9dc4-0355f38e006d/Presentation/PublicationAttachment/006a3453-d8c7-480a-8ba2-0857b3c08e74/LaborLaw10-Ch20.pdf. Accessed December 13, 2011.

2010 Nurse Alliance Quality Committees Program (2010). Available at: http://www.seiu.org/a/about-the-seiu-nurse-alliance.php. Accessed November 7, 2010.

Who we are, NNU (2010). Available at: http://www.nationalnursesunited.org/about/who-we-are.html. Accessed November 20, 2010.

STUDENT WORKBOOK ACTIVITY 8.1

Complete the following case scenarios based on the information provided in this chapter. You must use two vocabulary or key terms discussed in the text in each of your four answers. You can repeat two terms once.

Real-Life Applications: Case Scenario 1

You were just hired by a hospital as a replacement for a nurse manager that had recently quit. Working conditions are poor, and nurses are very upset about the number of patients assigned to each of them during a shift. You hear talk of nurses trying to organize a union that you know nothing about. The human resources manager provides information about how unions are formed.

Activity

Based on this information, create a checklist for union formation.

Responses

_____

_____

_____

_____

_____

Real-Life Applications: Case Scenario 2

You are a surgery resident in a hospital. You believe that your shifts are very long, which can influence the quality of care you are providing your patients. You do not know where or who to complain to. Your friend tells you that he and several other residents are interested in forming a union. You did not realize there was a union that would represent residents. You thought you were not eligible.

Activity

Based on your research, describe the union options available to residents.

_____

_____

_____

_____

_____

Real-Life Applications: Case Scenario 3

You were just hired as a health services administrator for a healthcare system. You have been hearing rumblings that the nurses and physicians who are employees would like to organize a union because management has not been responsive to their complaints. You did not realize that there were unions that represent both of these professionals.

Activity

Perform research and describe both nurses and physicians unions.

Responses

_____

_____

_____

_____

_____

Real-Life Applications: Case Scenario 4

With the continued focus on managed care, your employees are worried that focusing on cost cutting will reduce the quality of patient care. As a health services administrator, you are worried about the continued dissatisfaction.

Activity

Develop three strategies that would motivate and increase employee satisfaction.

Responses

_____

_____

_____

_____

_____

STUDENT WORKBOOK ACTIVITY 8.2

In Your Own Words

Please describe these core concepts in your own words.

Labor unions:

_____

_____

_____

_____

Grievance procedures:

_____

_____

_____

_____

Collective bargaining:

_____

_____

_____

_____

Alternative dispute resolution:

_____

_____

_____

_____

Bargaining unit:

_____

_____

_____

_____

Taft–Hartley Act:

_____

_____

_____

_____

Union authorization cards:

_____

_____

_____

_____

National Labor Relations Act:

_____

_____

_____

_____

Conciliation:

_____

_____

_____

_____

Arbitration:

_____

_____

_____

_____

STUDENT WORKBOOK ACTIVITY 8.3

Internet Exercises

Write your answers in the spaces provided.

- Visit each of the websites that are listed in the text that follows.
- Name the organization.
- Locate its mission statement on its website. If the organization does not have a mission statement, describe its purpose.
- Provide a brief overview of the activities of the organization.
- Apply this organization to the chapter information.

Websites

http://www.fmcs.gov

Organization name:

_____

Mission statement:

_____

_____

_____

Overview of activities:

_____

_____

_____

Application to chapter information:

_____

_____

_____

http://www.seiu.org

Organization name:

_____

Mission statement:

_____

_____

_____

Overview of activities:

_____

_____

_____

Application to chapter information:

_____

_____

_____

http://www.nlrb.gov

Organization name:

_____

Mission statement:

_____

_____

_____

Overview of activities:

_____

_____

_____

Application to chapter information:

_____

_____

_____

http://www.nationalnursesunited.org

Organization name:

_____

Mission statement:

_____

_____

_____

Overview of activities:

_____

_____

_____

Application to chapter information:

_____

_____

_____

http://www.nber.org
Organization name:

_____

Mission statement:

_____

_____

_____

Overview of activities:

_____

_____

_____

Application to chapter information:

_____

_____

_____

http://www.aft.org
Organization name:

_____

Mission statement:

_____

_____

_____

Overview of activities:

_____

_____

_____

Application to chapter information:

_____

_____

_____

STUDENT ACTIVITY 8.4: DISCUSSION BOARDS FOR ONLINE, HYBRID, AND TRADITIONAL ONGROUND CLASSES

Discussion Board Guidelines

The discussion board is used in online and web-enhanced courses in place of classroom lectures and discussion. The board can be an enhancement to traditional onground classes. The discussion board is the way in which the students "link together" as a class. The following are guidelines to help focus on the discussion topic and to define the roles and responsibilities of the discussion coordinator and other members of the class. The educator will be the discussion moderator for this course.

1. The educator will post the discussion topic and directions for the upcoming week. These postings should all be responses to the original topic or responses to other students' responses. When people respond to what someone else has posted, they should start the posting with the person's name so it is clear which

message they are responding to. **A response such as "Yes" or "I agree" does not count for credit. Your responses must be in your own words. You cannot copy and paste from the text.**

2. Postings (especially responses) should include enough information so the message is clear but should not be so long that it becomes difficult to follow. Remember, this is like talking to someone in a classroom setting. The postings should reflect the content of the textbook or other assignments. If you retrieve information from the Internet, the hyperlink must be cited.

3. Students should check the discussion daily to see if new information has been posted that requires their attention and response.

Good discussion will often include different points of view. Students should feel free to disagree or "challenge" others to support their positions or ideas. All discussions must be handled in a respectful manner. The following are discussion boards for this chapter.

Discussion Boards

1. What is a labor union? Do you agree or disagree with its purpose? Defend your answer.
2. Discuss the role labor unions have in the nursing sector of health care. Do you know any nurses that belong to a union?
3. Do you think physicians should have unions? Why or why not?
4. Define procedural justice. How does that relate to unions?

Terminating Healthcare Employees

The student will be able to:

- Illustrate the difference between employee dismissal and employee discharge.
- Identify the exceptions to employment-at-will doctrines.
- Assess alternative dispute resolution methods.
- Discuss the steps in the progressive discipline approach.
- Identify the difference between involuntary termination and administrative termination.
- Evaluate the importance of the employee handbook.

DID YOU KNOW THAT?

- Most states adhere to the employment-at-will doctrine, which means that in the absence of a legal employment contract, employees and employers can end their relationship for any reason.
- Termination of an employee is one of the most disliked responsibilities of supervisors in an organization.
- Employee handbooks have been upheld in court as being employment contracts.
- Employment practices liability insurance covers legal fees and settlement fees for organizations.
- A positive discipline approach consists of several conferences that focus on changing employee behavior from negative to positive.

■ Introduction

Employment is a relationship between an employee and an employer with expectations by each that the responsibilities of the other will be fulfilled. Both employers and employees have rights and should treat each other respectfully. Employers must provide a safe working environment for their employees. Employees must perform to the best of their ability in accordance with their job descriptions, which is why they were hired. However, that does not always happen; therefore there are laws and rules and regulations in place to ensure that both sides maintain their rights when an employee is terminated. The author decided to focus one chapter of this text solely on employee termination because it is often the most difficult action taken in an organization. Although this is the shortest chapter in the text, it may be the most important. If an organization has a legally defensible hiring process that provides an opportunity to hire the best employees for the organization, there should be minimal need to terminate many employees. If an employee is terminated for poor performance, it is possible that the person should not have been hired. The organization must emphasize to their employees that the hiring process must be a quality process that will select the best employees for an organization. In a recent survey of healthcare managers, healthcare employee terminations occurred for the following six reasons: (1) poor performance, (2) ethical misconduct, (3) inconsistent attendance, (4) poor attitude, (5) personality conflicts, and (6) substance abuse (McKinnies, Collins, Collins & Matthews, 2010). The primary reason termination occurred was poor performance by employees. Theoretically, routine feedback and discipline can change employee performance. However, termination occurs because some employees cannot change their performance.

There are two types of employee separation: employee dismissal and employee discharge. **Employee dismissal** occurs when an employee has not improved problems with job performance. **Employee discharge** occurs when an employee exhibits behavioral problems that are offenses for termination (Fallon & McConnell, 2007a).

The organization must impose discipline; if it does not, this may encourage other employees to exhibit similar negative behavior. If an organization allows negative behavior, it is supporting that behavior. Typically, an organization will have a progressive discipline process that consists of written warnings and eventual termination. All documented warnings are placed in the employee's personnel file. Initially, the supervisor may provide counsel to the employee. This also should be documented.

The passage of labor laws and the institution of unions have focused on establishing and enforcing employee rights in all aspects of their employment. This chapter will focus on employees' legal and contractual rights in the termination process, the impact of the employment-at-will doctrine on termination of employees, employee discipline approaches, and the importance of a systematic termination process.

■ Employment at Will

Most states adhere to the **employment-at-will doctrine**, which means that, in the absence of a legal employment contract, employees and employers can end their relationship for any reason. Employment-at-will policies are more prevalent in private organizations than public organizations. Local and federal laws protect public employees, and, depending on the state, a written notice of disciplinary action or a hearing for termination for cause is provided (Fried & Fottler, 2009). However, states vary as to what degree they support an employer's right to terminate employees under the employment-at-will doctrine: 43 states acknowledge the public-policy exception, 42 states acknowledge implied contract, and 20 states acknowledge breach of implied covenant of good faith and fair dealing (Employment at Will States, 2011). Approximately 55% of private employers operate an employment-at-will practice (Radin & Werhane, 2003). An example of a private employer using an employment-at-will doctrine is the firing of employees who smoke. Weyco, a medical benefits provider, banned employees from smoking outside workplace premises. Employees are subjected to random tests and have to agree to searches of personal belongings if officials suspect tobacco is being brought to the workplace (Trend: You Smoke? You're Fired, 2005).

■ Employment-at-Will Exceptions

There are three major exceptions to employment-at-will policies: implied contracts, the public-policy exception, and breach of implied covenant of good faith and fair dealing. **Implied contracts** can occur when a potential employer makes a verbal promise such as "if you do a great job, you will have a job for life" to an employee or an employee handbook or manual suggests a type of contract. If an employee handbook has a list of offenses that constitute termination for just cause, a court may assume that these offenses are the only reason an employee can be terminated, which invalidates employment at will. Therefore, it is important that the employee handbook have a disclaimer indicating it is not an implied contract for employees (Dalglish, 2000).

The **public-policy exception** states that an employer cannot terminate an employee if the employee refuses to comply with an employer's request to perform an illegal action that would violate a public policy, such as refusing to cover up Occupational Safety and Health Administration (OSHA) violations. If an employer fires an employee for refusing to violate public policy, this would be construed as **wrongful discharge**.

Finally, the **breach of implied covenant of good faith and fair dealing** has been adopted into the Uniform Commercial Code and the American Law Institute's Restatement of Contracts. It is the basic assumption of contractual relations that both parties will act fairly and in good faith (Dessler, 2011). Suppose an employer fires a long-term employee without cause, claiming employment at will. However, the long-term employee worked for the company under the assumption that if he performed to the best of his ability, he would be allowed to work for the company until his retirement. This could be a breach of good faith by the employer.

■ Due Process Methods

An alternative to employment-at-will doctrines is the establishment of **due process methods** that provide employees with the opportunity to appeal the organization's decision to terminate the employee. Due process also includes the fairness of the employer process of determining employee actions that result in disciplinary actions. Establishing these types of policies may avoid a legal dispute between the employee and employer. An alternative to arguing disciplinary actions in the court systems is **alternative dispute resolution methods,** which consist of open door policy, peer review panels mediation, and arbitration (Dessler, 2012).

An **open door policy,** the "in-house" method of resolving employment issues, is the easiest form of alternative dispute resolution. Supervisors indicate that if there are any employment issues, their door is open to any employee to discuss any potential problems from the employee's perspective. An employer should have a forum for disgruntled employees. An open door policy is the easiest method of providing an avenue for discussion. The disadvantage of an open door policy is that there is only one person, a supervisor, who is listening to an employee issue. The employee issue may be related to another supervisor who is friendly with the employee supervisor that is listening to employee complaints. However, rather than having no due process in place, an open door policy can be beneficial to both the employee and the employer. A second in-house method is peer review panels. **Peer review panels** consist of specially trained employees that become involved in evaluating employee disputes. They are required to sign confidentiality agreements regarding the process. They review the dispute and make recommendations to resolve the dispute, which both sides agree to follow.

Two external procedures for resolving employment disputes are mediation and arbitration. Unlike the open door policy and peer review panels, both mediation and arbitration use an external third party to hear the complaint. **Mediation** is also a third-party system but with less rigidity. The mediator intercedes to resolve a dispute, but the mediator's suggested agreement is not legally binding (Dessler, 2011). **Arbitration** uses a third-party system to make a decision regarding the employment dispute. The decision of the arbitrator is a binding decision that both parties must abide by and is enforceable under federal and state laws.

The **American Arbitration Association** (AAA), which is the largest alternative dispute resolution provider, trains individuals in resolving employment issues through arbitration and mediation. Established in 1926, this nonprofit public organization has been responsible for dispute resolutions in many different industries including health care. In 2001, AAA launched the Healthcare Payer Provider Arbitration Rules, which focuses on reimbursement disputes between providers and payers in the healthcare industry (About Us, 2011).

The United States is a litigious society. In addition to establishing alternative dispute resolution methods, organizations including healthcare organization are purchasing insurance to protect them from numerous lawsuits. **Employment practices liability insurance** (EPLI) covers employer legal fees, settlements, and judgments due to employment matters. These insurance products became popular in the 1990s when the Civil Rights Act of 1991 (amendment to the Civil Rights Act of 1964) was passed, which allowed financial damages for discrimination and harassment suits. There are currently 60 carriers for EPLI that cover all industries including the healthcare industry (What Is EPLI?, 2011).

■ Employee Discipline

Termination of employment is the result of unacceptable behavior by the employee as determined by organizational policy, procedures, and ultimately employment law. Organizations must have a system in place to discipline employees in order for employees to understand if their behavior is positive or negative. Employees who exhibit negative behavior that does not receive feedback do not understand or know that their behavior is, in fact, negative. Most employers use the progressive discipline approach, which is a formal discipline process in which repeated negative behavior results in more serious disciplinary measures. The following are typical steps in a **progressive discipline approach** (Byars & Rue, 2006):

1. Oral warning: often unofficial between supervisor and employee.
2. Official written warning: goes in personnel file.
3. Second written warning: could also include temporary suspension threat.
4. Temporary suspension plus notice of possible termination.
5. Termination.

Establishing a progressive discipline approach depends on the organization's diligence in written policies and procedures for employee performance and expectations. Another popular disciplinary approach is the **positive discipline approach,** which assumes that employees can change their behavior if given constructive criticism. The approach consists of problem-solving conferences between the employee and supervisor. The four steps of the positive discipline approach include:

1. Counseling: Inform employee of organizational rules. This is a conference between the supervisor and the employee.
2. Written documentation: The employee fails to correct behavior after step 1, and written documentation is noted in the employee's personnel file. The conference result is written up and placed in the employee's personnel file.
3. Final warning: A conference is held, and the employee is asked to develop an action plan to remedy inappropriate behavior. This is placed in the employee's personnel file.
4. Termination: If the action plan is not followed, then the employee will be terminated (Dessler, 2011).

Many supervisors are uncomfortable with these processes. Disciplining employees can be difficult particularly in a small organization where socializing is common among employees. However, negative employee behavior must have ramifications or more employees will exhibit similar behavior, assuming that it is acceptable. To increase the supervisor's comfort level, training supervisors should receive training regarding these disciplinary processes.

■ Involuntary Termination of an Employee

An employer initiates **involuntary termination** of an employee. It is a difficult process to initiate and rarely a happy occasion for either the employer or employee. It is extremely important that there is a written process in place to document this decision because of potential lawsuits that may be initiated by the unhappy employee. Employees are terminated **for cause**, which occurs when an employee jeopardizes other employees. Examples are stealing or threatening another employee. This may be the easiest way to terminate an employee because the action is an open violation of company policies. Employees can be terminated because of poor work performance. This reason is typically documented, as the employee with poor performance will have received documentation on how to improve. The employee is terminated if the performance does not improve. A more difficult termination is an **administrative termination**, which means it is a termination of employment without cause, such as a layoff of employees. Layoffs occur because there has been a downturn in the performance of the company or in the economy that results in less need for labor or because technology has eliminated positions, also resulting in less need for labor. This type of termination is not the fault of the employee typically; therefore, it is more difficult for the employee to accept. This type of termination does allow the company to rehire the employee if needed at a future date. The employee can collect unemployment benefits (Hume, 2011).

■ Importance of the Employee Handbook

When the new employee is hired, one of the first pieces of documentation given to the individual is an **employee handbook**. This handbook is a guide for the employee to the organization's expectations of employee behavior. It also is a guide to the policies and procedures of the organization. During orientation, the employer reviews the handbook with the employee. When a new employee is given a copy of the handbook, the organization should also ask that the employee sign a receipt indicating he or she has received it, maintaining the receipt in the employee personnel file. All employees should have a copy of the handbook. Supervisors should be very familiar with its content. If there are any changes to the handbook during the tenure of an employee, all updated handbook information must be given to the employee with an additional signed statement by the employee that the updates were provided. This procedure eliminates any claims that an employee was not familiar with the policies and procedures of the handbook. To avoid the impression that a handbook is an employee contract, the handbook is written objectively, providing facts about organizational procedures. There should be no guarantees or promises regarding employment. Even if organizations include a disclaimer that the handbook is not an employment contract, some courts have ruled that a handbook could be construed as an employment contract. To avoid this issue, Fallon and McConnell (2007b) suggest that a new employee who is considered temporary or probationary and has passed the probationary period should be considered a regular employee, not a permanent employee, because the description "permanent employee" may lead the employee to believe he or she is immune to termination.

■ A Checklist for Terminating Employees

Termination of an employee is one of the most difficult processes in an organization. The process must be legally defensible to ensure the liability protection of the organization. Lawsuits for wrongful discharge can be very expensive to an organization. Lynott (2004), Perry (1997), Steingold (2004), and this author have identified a checklist to ensure that the process is fair and legal:

1. Employee education on employment law and company policies: Both supervisors and their employees should receive training regarding their rights in an organization. The training will help both parties to understand their obligations to the organization and the organization's legal obligation to them.
2. Communication: Communicate both verbally and in writing the expectations the organization has of the employee's performance. Communication begins during the hiring process with the job description. Routine communication continues throughout the employment, documenting any issues with the employee's performance and communicating these issues to the employee. The communications must be maintained in the personnel file of the employee. When the employee is terminated, a termination letter should be given to the employee detailing the reasons why the employee is terminated.
3. Consistency: Enforcement of labor laws equally applied to all employees to ensure there are no issues with discrimination of protected classes.
4. Routine performance appraisals: Establish routine performance appraisals of all employees. These appraisals should be standard and applied to all employees.
5. Employee feedback: During any performance appraisal process, allow an opportunity for the employee to review the evaluation, to make comments, and to initial documentation that they acknowledge and understand the evaluation.
6. Termination deadline: Because employee termination can be a very difficult situation, employers may continue to allow a poor performer to continue in an organization. Establishing a time frame for employee dismissal supports the legal defensibility of the termination process.

7. Exit interview: Managers should have an exit interview with the terminated employee in a comfortable environment. Treat the employee with respect. Do not e-mail their termination letter prior to the interview. Discuss the specific reasons why the employee is terminated, giving him or her a termination letter detailing the reasons. If possible, provide some placement counseling for the terminated employee, discussing his or her future elsewhere. Have his or her final paycheck ready if possible. If there is a potential for litigation, have another individual present who could be a witness to the interview process.
8. Confidentiality: Do not discuss the termination exit interview with other employees. This will prevent any possibilities of lawsuits by the terminated employee for defamation.

This checklist should provide guidelines to ensure that a termination process is fair to the employee, which should avoid any litigation.

■ Conclusion

Termination of an employee is one of the most difficult responsibilities for a manager because it affects the individual's livelihood. If you have to terminate an employee, it may indicate that the organization's hiring process is not adequate. Many guidelines should be followed to ensure that the termination process is legally defensible while providing interactional justice to the employee who is being terminated.

■ Vocabulary

Administrative termination
Alternative dispute resolution
  methods
American Arbitration Association
Arbitration
Breach of implied covenant of good
  faith and fair dealing
Due process methods
Employee discharge
Employee dismissal
Employee handbook
Employment practices liability
  insurance

Employment-at-will doctrine
For cause
Implied contracts
Involuntary termination
Mediation
Open door policy
Peer review panels
Positive discipline approach
Progressive discipline approach
Public-policy exception
Wrongful discharge

■ References

About Us (2011). Available at: http://www.adr.org/about. Accessed July 15, 2011.

Byars, L. & Rue, L. (2006). *Human Resource Management* (8th ed.). New York, NY: McGraw-Hill/ Irwin, pp. 355–360.

Dalglish, R. (2000). Avoiding the legal pitfalls of hiring and firing. *JCK*, June: 306–313.

Dessler, G. (2011). *A Framework for Human Resource Management*. Upper Saddle River, NJ: Prentice Hall, pp. 273–280.

Dessler, G. (2012). *Fundamentals of Human Resource Management*. Upper Saddle River, NJ: Prentice Hall, pp. 295–300.

Employment at Will States (2011). Available at: http://employeeissues.com/at_will_states.html. Accessed March 20, 2011.

Fallon, L. & McConnell, C. (2007a). *Human Resource Management in Health Care*. Sudbury, MA: Jones & Bartlett, pp. 247–276.

Fallon, L. & McConnell, C. (2007b). *Human Resource Management In Health Care*. Sudbury, MA: Jones & Bartlett, pp. 304–305.

Fried, B. & Fottler, M. (2008). *Human Resources in Healthcare* (3rd ed.). Chicago, IL: Health Administration Press, p. 135.

Hume, J. (2011). What is considered an administrative termination of employment? Available at: http:// www.ehow.com/print/facts_6743680_considered-administrative-termination-employment. Accessed March 20, 2011.

Lynott, W. (2004). How to Discharge an Employee & Stay out of Trouble Doing It. Available at: http:// restaurant-hospitality.com/features/rh_imp_5831/. Accessed January 1, 2012.

McKinnies, R., Collins, S., Collins, K. & Matthews, E. (2010). Lack of performance: The top reasons for terminating healthcare employees. *Journal of Radiology Management*, 32(3):44–47.

Perry, P. (1997). How to terminate employees without landing in court. *Materials Management in Healthcare*, 97(6):1–6.

Radin, T. & Werhane, P. (2003). Employment at will, employee rights, and future directions for employment. *Business Ethics Quarterly*, 13(2):113–130.

Steingold, F. (2004). Firing employees and avoiding trouble. *American Coin-Op*, 45(2):1–3.

Trend: You Smoke? You're Fired. (2005). *USA Today*, May 12.

What Is EPLI? (2011). Available at: http://www.iii.org/individuals/business/optional/epli/. Accessed July 16, 2011.

STUDENT WORKBOOK ACTIVITY 9.1

Complete the following case scenarios based on the information provided in this chapter. You must use two vocabulary or key terms discussed in the text in each of your four answers. You can repeat two terms once.

Real-Life Applications: Case Scenario 1

You were just appointed to a management position. One of your first tasks is to review all of the employees in your department and assess their performance. It is your understanding there are two employees who need to be disciplined.

Activity

Define the different approaches to disciplining your employees. Select the progressive discipline approach and explain how you will apply it to your employees.

Responses

_____

_____

_____

_____

_____

Real-Life Applications: Case Scenario 2

Your employer has recently been sued by two employees for wrongful termination. The lawyer for your healthcare facility indicates that it is necessary to revamp the termination procedures.

Activity

Develop a checklist for an employee termination procedure.

Responses

_____

_____

_____

_____

_____

Real-Life Applications: Case Scenario 3

You just bought a skilled nursing facility. After reviewing its employee policies and procedures, you realized that the employees were not aware of these policies.

Activity

Discuss the importance of an employee handbook and the role it can play in employee terminations.

Responses

_____

_____

_____

_____

_____

Real-Life Applications: Case Scenario 4

As a new nurse manager, you have opted to select the positive discipline approach to managing employee behaviors.

Activity

List the steps in the positive discipline approach and explain how you would apply it to the nurses that you supervise.

Responses

_____

_____

_____

_____

_____

STUDENT WORKBOOK ACTIVITY 9.2

In Your Own Words

Please describe these core concepts in your own words.

Employment at will:

_____

_____

_____

_____

Administrative termination:

_____

_____

_____

_____

Involuntary termination:

_____

_____

_____

_____

Employee dismissal:

_____

_____

_____

_____

Employee discharge:

_____

_____

_____

_____

Due process methods:

_____

_____

_____

_____

Public-policy exception:

_____

_____

_____

_____

Alternative dispute resolution methods:

_____

_____

_____

_____

Peer review panels:

_____

_____

_____

_____

Arbitration:

_____

_____

_____

_____

STUDENT WORKBOOK ACTIVITY 9.3

Internet Exercises

Write your answers in the spaces provided.

- Visit each of the websites that are listed in the text that follows.
- Name the organization.
- Locate its mission statement on its website. If the organization does not have a mission statement, describe its purpose.
- Provide a brief overview of the activities of the organization.
- Apply this organization to the chapter information.

Websites
www.adr.org

Organization name:

_____

Mission statement:

_____

_____

_____

Overview of activities:

_____

_____

_____

Application to chapter information:

_____

_____

_____

http://www.employeeissues.com

Organization name:

_____

Mission statement:

_____

_____

_____

Overview of activities:

_____

_____

_____

Application to chapter information:

_____

_____

_____

http://www.iii.org

Organization name:

_____

Mission statement:

_____

_____

_____

Overview of activities:

_____

_____

_____

Application to chapter information:

_____

_____

_____

http://www.nfib.com

Organization name:

_____

Mission statement:

_____

_____

_____

Overview of activities:

_____

_____

_____

Application to chapter information:

_____

_____

_____

http://www.healthlawyers.org

Organization name:

_____

Mission statement:

_____

_____

_____

Overview of activities:

_____

_____

_____

Application to chapter information:

_____

_____

_____

http://www.hg.org
Organization name:

_____

Mission statement:

_____

_____

_____

Overview of activities:

_____

_____

_____

Application to chapter information:

_____

_____

_____

STUDENT ACTIVITY 9.4: DISCUSSION BOARDS FOR ONLINE, HYBRID, AND TRADITIONAL ONGROUND CLASSES

Discussion Board Guidelines

The discussion board is used in online and web-enhanced courses in place of classroom lectures and discussion. The board can be an enhancement to traditional classes. The discussion board is the way in which the students "link together" as a class. The following are guidelines to help focus on the discussion topic and to define the roles and responsibilities of the discussion coordinator and other members of the class. The educator will be the discussion moderator for this course.

1. The educator will post the discussion topic and directions for the upcoming week. These postings should all be responses to the original topic or responses to other students' responses. When people respond to what someone else has posted, they should start the posting with the person's name so it is clear which message they are responding to. **A response such as "Yes" or "I agree" does not count for credit. Your responses must be in your own words. You cannot copy and paste from the text.**
2. Postings (especially responses) should include enough information so the message is clear but should not be so long that it becomes difficult to follow. Remember, this is like talking to someone in a classroom setting. The postings should reflect the content of the text or other assignments. If you retrieve information from the Internet, the hyperlink must be cited.
3. Students should check the discussion daily to see if new information has been posted that requires their attention and response.

Good discussion will often include different points of view. Students should feel free to disagree or "challenge" others to support their positions or ideas. All discussions must be handled in a respectful manner. The following are discussion boards for this chapter.

Discussion Boards

1. Which do think is more affective? Positive discipline or progressive discipline approach? Defend your answer.
2. How do you feel about employment at will policies? Are they fair?
3. Discuss the different types of due process approaches. What experiences have you had with these approaches.
4. Perform an internet search. Discuss a company that uses EPLI.

Long-Term Planning in HR

Current Trends in Healthcare Human Resource Management

DID YOU KNOW THAT?

- The basic form of telemedicine is a telephone consultation.
- Effective teamwork in patient care can improve the quality of care.
- The U.S. Department of Defense and the Agency for Healthcare Research and Quality have formed a national training initiative for healthcare professionals.
- The federal government is encouraging the use of electronic prescriptions for Medicare patients by paying bonuses to providers.
- In the 1950s, medical faculty at an American university developed a problem-based learning format to encourage teamwork in health care.

■ Introduction

The diversity of the healthcare workforce, healthcare globalization, use of technology, the focus on teamwork in patient care, accountable care organizations, the pay for performance model, and use of social media as a communication tool are current trends in health care that affect healthcare human resource management (HRM).

The diversity of employees and of patients in the United States is increasing. The U.S. Census Bureau projects that the Asian and Hispanic populations will both triple and the African-American population will double by 2050 (Salisbury & Byrd, 2006). Through 2050, there will be U.S. healthcare labor shortages with serious shortages in remote and rural areas resulting in the hiring of international employees (What's Different About Rural Health Care?, 2011). More U.S. patients are seeking healthcare services internationally because of the high costs of U.S. health care. Healthcare service delivery is affected by the use of technology. The implementation of electronic health records has increased nationally. The focus on teamwork in health care is a new trend. Use of social media as a communication and education tool is a future trend. Each of these initiatives requires HRM training and development. In addition to these trends, the formation of Accountable Care Organizations (ACOs) requires orientation of employees to a new organizational structure. This chapter will describe these trends and the role that HRM plays in this changing environment.

■ Increasing Diversity in the Healthcare Workforce

Workplace diversity can be defined as an environment that recognizes the unique contributions that individuals with many types of differences can make (Diversity in the Workplace, 2011). Traditionally, males have dominated management positions. Women and minorities have been underrepresented in senior healthcare management. In a recent survey by the American College of Healthcare Executives (ACHE), women employees were more likely to serve as department heads and men were more likely to serve as CEOs, presidents, or vice presidents. Over a 15-year period of ACHE surveys, the proportion of women and other protected classes that were promoted to senior management did not significantly increase (Women in Healthcare Administration, 2011). The ACHE has recommended the following actions to correct this prevailing situation:

1. Develop promotion policies that focus on promoting a qualified diverse workforce.
2. Routinely review salaries of senior management to ensure there is no discrimination.
3. Review the organization's mission and vision statements for its focus on diversity.
4. Survey employees regarding diversity issues in the workplace, and routinely provide educational programs for employees regarding attitudes toward diversity (Gathers, 2003).

These actions can be implemented in collaboration with the human resources (HR) department and senior management. For the first two recommendations, HR can provide metrics for each policy such as number of women in senior management positions and the number of other protected classes in senior management positions. These metrics can be measured with historical data to observe any positive trends. For the last two recommendations, in conjunction with HR, senior management should work with all levels of employees to review the mission and vision statement and to implement the survey.

Cultural Competency Model

Another way to increase diversity in health care is the development of a cultural competency model. In 2002, the Institute of Medicine issued a report indicating that minority patients often received a lower quality of care in the U.S. system. New initiatives were taken to address these issues; however, in 2007 the **National Healthcare Disparities Report** indicated that the disparities had not greatly improved (Clark, 2006). In 2009, the **Joint Commission** and the **National Committee on Quality Assurance** began to develop standards for healthcare organizations to create a culturally sensitive environment for both employees and healthcare consumers. It has been documented that there is greater mistrust of healthcare providers among minority patients. This could in part be the result of lack of communication due to language barriers or low literacy. The issue of language barriers could have adverse outcomes for medical care (Andrulis, 2003). Betancourt, Green, Carrillo, and Ananeh-Firempong II (2003) defined the concept of **cultural competency** as the healthcare system's ability to provide patients quality care that is tailored to meet their social, cultural, and language needs. In 2006, Lehigh Valley Health Network, located in Allentown, Pennsylvania, implemented an organization-wide cultural competency model to produce equitable care to its patients. Its patient base encompassed urban, suburban, and rural communities that included Latino, Middle Eastern, and Southeast Asian populations. Prior to its cultural awareness project, the network's diversity initiatives were limited and showed mixed results. This new project was supported by senior leadership and implemented by the HR department. Other healthcare facilities that have developed a cultural competency model include White Memorial Medical Center in Los Angeles, California; Kaiser Permanente in San Francisco, California; and Sunset Park Family Health Center at Lutheran Medical Center in Brooklyn, New York (Betancourt, Green & Carrillo, 2002).

Gertner et al. (2010) and Hunt (2007) developed the following guidelines to create a **culturally competent healthcare organization:**

1. **Strategic cultural plan:** The organization must review its strategic plan and include a mission and vision statement that addresses diversity in the organization.
2. Standardized patient data collection: Patient registration is standardized to ensure patient demographic data are routinely collected.
3. Baseline employee survey: Prior to project implementation, surveys are given to assess baseline cultural awareness by employees.

4. Education program: Based on these employee surveys, an educational program is developed to address any employee weaknesses regarding cultural awareness. Part of the education program includes language assistance services to assist with translation, if needed.
5. Recruitment of diverse employees: Hiring diverse employees creates an environment of cultural acceptance of healthcare consumers.
6. Cultural materials: Culturally appropriate multimedia materials are developed and distributed to the network for both employees and consumers.
7. Systematic implementation: The organization must embrace these changes at all levels. Any changes are reviewed annually to ensure cultural competency.
8. Employee performance measurements: Include employee performance measurements to ensure cultural competency is maintained.

An organizational-wide initiative for cultural diversity provides a sustainable organizational culture. As the United States becomes more culturally diverse, healthcare systems need to reflect the values, beliefs, and behaviors of patients (Betancourt et al., 2002). Achieving cultural competency promotes equitable health care. Diversity in the workplace is a necessity because patient diversity has increased. Patients are more comfortable seeking health care from an individual who is similar to them in ethnicity, age, or gender, so it is important for models such as the cultural competency model and the ACHE recommendations to be implemented to increase diversity.

■ Healthcare Globalization

Medical Tourism

The **globalization of healthcare** has occurred because of the diversity in both employees and healthcare consumers and the increase in services being offered outside the United States as an alternative to costly U.S. medical procedures. More countries have developed medical expertise to provide healthcare services at a much lower cost than in the United States. This phenomenon has developed into **medical tourism**, which means that patients opt to have medical procedures performed outside the United States because the cost is less while quality is maintained. Many U.S. patients seek international care because they are uninsured or underinsured. Most patients seek overseas care for dental, cosmetic, orthopedic, and cardiovascular services.

A recent McKinsey & Co. report indicated that in addition to cost savings, 40% of international patients seek advanced technological health care, 32% seek better healthcare services, and 15% seek faster medical care. In 2007, the number of U.S. patients seeking medical care overseas ranged from 500,000 to 750,000. The medical tourism market is currently a $20 billion market with projected increases to more than $100 billion within the next 5 years (Medical Tourism, 2011). According to a recent liver transplant patient, a U.S. hospital would have charged him $450,000 for the procedure, and that hospital could not schedule the procedure for months. He went to India and was charged $58,000, which included a 10-week hospital stay for both himself and his spouse (Ellis & Shanley, 2011).

According to a 2009 survey by the ACHE, the number of individuals who will travel for overseas medical treatments will double by 2014. This concept of medical tourism is becoming more popular because treatments provided outside the United States often cost one half or less than the cost of treatments provided in the United States (Pavarini, 2009). This movement of patients is becoming more common. There are several websites that promote medical tourism, such as www.medicaltourism.com and www.medretreat.com. Many Central and South American countries have strong reputations for elective surgeries. India is offering affordable high-quality care with prices 10% less than the cost of those in the United States. Thailand, Malaysia, and Singapore are popular for cardiac surgery (Horowitz, Rosensweig & Jones, 2007).

Because of this global trend, U.S. companies are now offering international medical packages for their employees because it is more cost effective. Basic Plus Health Insurance is offering its members an option of overseas care at hospitals accredited by the Joint Commission International. They entered into an agreement with Companion Global Healthcare, a medical tourism facilitator located in Columbia, South Carolina, to develop a network of approved services in foreign locations (Companion Global Healthcare, Inc., 2011).

Although the quality of international care continues to be debated, medical tourism continues to increase in popularity. Both the Joint Commission International and the International Organization for Standardization provide quality management services for global healthcare services. The Medical Tourism Association is a nonprofit membership organization that promotes quality of care and education regarding this type of health care (About Medical Tourism, 2012).

U.S. Healthcare Organizations Offer Overseas Services

In addition to foreign healthcare organizations offering more services to U.S. citizens, more U.S. healthcare organizations are now offering their healthcare services overseas. Managers, including HR managers, must continually address the following differences in international management (Byars & Rue, 2006):

1. Sociocultural: norms and values, religious beliefs, and educational levels that influence the delivery of healthcare services. Employees must be trained to ensure they understand the culture where they will be working. Religious beliefs may affect how workdays are structured. Educational levels are very important to understand for hiring purposes. If the educational level is not appropriate, then the organization should not be located in that country.

2. Economic: wage levels, per capita income, and monetary policies. In particular, wage levels and per capita income are important for the organization to know so that it can pay host country nationals appropriately.
3. Politico-legal: tax laws, government policies, stability of government. The stability of the government and the relationship the host government has with the United States is very important. In addition, how the government views the healthcare organization is also vital to establishing a quality workforce and a quality environment for employees.

All of these factors influence the operations of organizations, including healthcare organizations. It is important to recognize and respect the differences in cultures. For example, organizations may hire **host country nationals** (HCNs), which are citizens of the country where the organization will be located. HCNs can provide insight into how to hire local employees and how to manage the organization within the cultural realm of the country. A healthcare organization may collaborate with a local healthcare organization. This may encourage acceptance of the foreign healthcare system.

The **Cleveland Clinic** is an example of a global healthcare system. Originally established in Cleveland, Ohio, its strategic plan targeted its services to the surrounding suburbs. The Cleveland Clinic currently operates 15 family health centers, which also contain pharmacies, and outpatient surgery centers in those areas. However, recognizing the need to increase its exposure nationally and internationally, the Cleveland Clinic established healthcare facilities in Weston, Florida; West Palm Beach, Florida; and Toronto, Canada, in 1988 and is scheduled to open a healthcare facility in Abu Dhabi, United Arab Emirates, in 2012. Cleveland Clinic Toronto has a facility for secondary and tertiary care and a wellness center. This was the result of a drop in treating overseas patients. The newest facility, Cleveland Clinic Abu Dhabi, will be a 360-bed multispecialty facility. The Cleveland Clinic negotiated a 15-year contract to construct, staff, and manage this hospital in the United Arab Emirates. The Cleveland Clinic also negotiated a similar arrangement in Vienna, Austria, and will be building a cardiac hospital in Shanghai, China. In these instances, the Cleveland Clinic will not own the hospitals but will manage them. To maintain the integrity of Cleveland Clinic's quality patient care, all of the facilities will be staffed by Cleveland Clinic physicians. The Cleveland Clinic is currently recruiting for U.S. citizens to work at the United Arab Emirates site (Staff Qualifications, 2011). Recently, **Duke University Health Systems** signed a 7-year agreement with Peking University to improve the healthcare systems in China. Duke University Health Systems will develop joint research, specialty clinical care programs, and management training (Ellis & Shanley, 2011).

■ Technology

The Institute of Medicine (IOM) has published reports over the past several years that focus on improving the quality of health care in the United States. In 2001, it published the report *Crossing the Quality Chasm: A New Health System for the 21st Century*, which stresses the importance of improving the Information Technology (IT) infrastructure. IOM emphasized the importance of an electronic health record (EHR), an electronic record of a patient's medical history. The report also described the importance of patient safety through establishment of data standards for collection of patient information (Institute of Medicine, 2001).

Because of these IOM reports, in 2004 President Bush established the **Office of the National Coordinator for Information Technology** within the U.S. Department of Health and Human Services. In 2005, the **American Health Information Community** (AHIC) was chartered to develop recommendations on how to increase health information technology (HIT) use in our healthcare system. AHIC focused on surveillance, consumer awareness, chronic health care, and EHRs. This federal advisory board concluded its work in 2008, and in the same year, this initiative was renamed the **National eHealth Collaborative**. This organization has already met with President Obama regarding HIT. During his tenure, President Bush indicated that most U.S. citizens should have an electronic patient record by 2014. President Obama has also supported this issue and has budgeted $19 billion to accelerate the use of computerized medical records in physicians' offices by creating regional HIT extension centers (Department of Health and Human Services, 2011). The American Recovery and Reinvestment Act of 2009 has allocated $20 billion for meaningful use of EHRs under the **Health Information Technology for Economic and Clinical Health Act of 2009**. **Meaningful use** has been identified by the federal government as using certified EHR technology for e-prescribing, exchanging electronic information for improving care, and submitting information to the federal government on clinical quality measures (Lamont, 2010). Incentive payments are made to providers that have at least 30 patients who are Medicare and Medicaid eligible.

Electronic Medical and Health Records

History

In 1991 and 1997, the IOM issued reports that focused on the impact of computer-based patients' records as an important technology for improving health care (Vreeman, Taggard, Rhine & Worrell, 2006). There are two concepts in electronic patient records that are used interchangeably but are different—the **electronic medical record** (EMR/EHR) and the **electronic health record** (EHR). The **National Alliance for Health Information Technology** (NAHIT) defines the EHR as the electronic record of health-related information on an individual that is accumulated from one health system and is used by the health organization that is providing patient care. The EMR accumulates patient medical information from the healthcare organizations that have been involved in the patient's care. Simply, the EHR is an EMR that can be integrated with other systems (National Alliance for Health Information Technology, 2008). The IOM has been urging the healthcare industry to adopt the electronic patient record, but initially costs were too high, and the health community did not embrace the recommendation. This discussion will focus on the EHR.

As software costs have declined, more healthcare providers have adopted the EHR system. In 2003, the U.S. Department of Health and Human Services began to promote the use of HIT including the use of the EHR. The IOM was asked to identify essential elements for the establishment of an EHR. The IOM broadly defined the definition of an EHR to include:

- The collection of longitudinal data on a person's health.
- Immediate electronic access to this information.
- Establishment of a system that provides decision support to ensure the quality, safety, and efficiency of patient care (Institute of Medicine, 2011).

Benefits of Electronic Medical Record/Electronic Health Record

Several studies have been performed to assess the impact of the EHR on healthcare delivery. Administrators of several healthcare delivery systems reported many benefits to the implementation of an EHR. Many administrators cited the capability of more comprehensive reporting that integrated both clinical and administrative data. The EHR also provided an opportunity to analyze and review patient outcomes because of the standardization of the clinical assessments. Also noted was the development of electronic automated reports that improved the discharge of patients. The reports also provided an opportunity for the administrator to assess the workload of a department. The EHR also improved operational efficiency. The EHR had excellent capabilities for processing and storage of data. Administrators also reported that the computerized documentation required 30% less time to complete than the previous handwritten notes (Shields et al., 2007). However, it is difficult to develop an electronic record that can integrate with other medical systems. It is important that standards be developed for the EHR to ensure standard data elements are collected and to ensure that the software will be integrated into other systems.

Several studies indicated that the EHR led to an improvement in interdepartmental communication. The EHR was used to provide aggregate data in patient records to various departments, and the information about the patients was legible. The actual design and implementation of an EHR system contributed to the development of a more interdisciplinary approach to patient care (Ventres & Shah, 2007; Whitman & David, 2007). The implementation of an EHR system led to improved data accuracy because it reduced the need to replicate data. The EHR system also provided a platform for routine data quality assessments, which was important to maintain the accuracy of the EHR data. The EHR system provides an opportunity for future research. The data captured in the database could be used to analyze outcomes and to develop baseline data for future research.

According to Valerius (2007), migration from a hard-copy system to an electronic system requires several components, including a physician order communication/results retrieval, electronic document/control management, point-of-care charting, electronic physician order entry and prescribing, clinical decision support system, provider patient portals, personal health records, and population health. When an organization implements an electronic system, there are changes in the workflow because much of the process was previously manual. Training is required for both healthcare professionals and staff to use the system.

When purchasing a system for patient electronic records, it had been found that there could be equipment or software inadequacies that caused slower processing of the data. If the system failed, it created frustration for healthcare professionals and administrators. Both of these problems emphasized the need for adequate training for both the providers and the staff. Much of the initial training required overtime for the staff. Most of the training lasted approximately 4 months. Continued training was also required for maintenance of a system (Valerius, 2007).

In October 2008, Microsoft announced its Health Vault website (Health Vault, 2012), which enables patients to develop EHRs free of charge. The individual chooses how much medical information to store online with this website. The website also has links to several health websites that provide information about exercise programs, heart issues, and drug reactions; provide software that allows users to share their medical information with their providers; and so forth. In November 2008, the Cleveland Clinic agreed to pilot data exchanges between Health Vault and the Cleveland Clinic's personal health record system. The clinic enrolled 250 patients in the areas of diabetes, hypertension, and heart disease to test the system. The patients tested their health status at home using blood pressure monitors, weight scales, heart rate monitors, and glucometers. These reports were uploaded to the Cleveland Clinic using Health Vault. The patients were able to access health education material on Health Vault regarding their diseases. This was the first pilot study in the country to assess this tool. The results of the pilot study indicated that there was a significant time difference between doctor visits by diabetic patients because patients had gained better control of their conditions. However, heart patients visited their physicians more often because of their self-testing, indicating more timely visiting. The patients felt more in control of their personal health and felt they were partners with their physicians regarding their care (Cleveland Clinic/Microsoft Pilot Promising, 2011).

Although these initiatives have been touted as progress in managing patients' care, the IOM recently issued a 2011 report indicating that these initiatives, although progressive, need to be closely monitored. The IOM recommended the establishment of a new governmental oversight agency for HIT efforts to ensure patient confidentiality.

In addition to the implementation of the EHR system itself, the new HIT agency must carefully monitor the EHR vendors that have developed software for healthcare organizations. Vendors have routinely hidden software errors that may have increased user error, such as a clinician misplacing decimal points for dosages because the keys on the keyboard are too close together, resulting in a patient hazard (Hirsch, 2011).

E-prescribing

Technology has greatly influenced how providers are ordering prescriptions. **E-prescribing** is electronic prescription ordering by a provider for a patient and improves patient safety. Medication ordering and the administration of medication can be faulty because of similar-sounding drug names, similar dosages, or similar labeling. E-prescribing can be performed on a desktop computer, laptop, or handheld device that will record a physician's prescription order, eliminating the need for an individual to read an illegible handwritten prescription. In January 2009, Medicare and some private healthcare plans began paying bonuses to physicians who e-prescribe medications for their Medicare patients. Medicare will penalize physicians who do not e-prescribe by 2012 by reducing their reimbursement rates by 1%. IT companies are providing free software to physicians to encourage them to electronically prescribe. The number of physicians who are e-prescribing has risen over the past year. It is estimated that between 12% and 16% of all office-based physicians are e-prescribing. E-prescribing encourages patients to fill their prescriptions because it reduces waiting times at the drugstore. A limitation with e-prescribing is that federal laws prohibit electronic prescribing of any type of controlled substance, which could include sleeping pills or antidepressant drugs (Landro, 2009). An e-prescribing system can be used alone, but it is best used with the EHR system because it integrates the information from the patient's EHR into its decision-making logic, further assisting healthcare providers with their patient care decisions.

The Clinical Decision Support Expert Review Panel recommended that an e-prescribing system contain the following database elements: patient payer and plan data, patient medications and their status, patient demographic information, patient allergies to drugs, diagnoses, laboratory tests, and pharmacy information. The panel also recommended that users should (1) be able to select dosage, strength, and duration; (2) be made aware of any drug alerts regarding drug interactions; (3) be able to view patient instructions; (4) be able to view weight-based dosing; (5) be able to view food interactions with drugs; (6) be notified when the prescription is due for renewal; and (7) be notified if the patient does not refill the prescription (Teich et al., 2005).

Telemedicine

Technology has improved how providers communicate with their patients. **Telemedicine** refers to the use of IT to enable healthcare providers to communicate with rural care providers regarding patient care or to communicate directly with patients regarding treatment. The basic form of telemedicine is a telephone consultation. Telemedicine is frequently used in pathology and radiology because images can be transmitted to a distant location where a specialist will read the results. Telemedicine is becoming more common because it increases healthcare access to remote locations such as rural areas. It also is a cost-effective mode of treatment. As EMRs/EHRs are used more frequently, it will be possible to provide services that are more comprehensive. A limitation may be how to reimburse a provider for providing an electronic consultation. Another limitation may also be if there are issues with reimbursement across state lines (Anderson, Rice & Kominski, 2007).

Robotic Surgery

Robots were first introduced as a surgical tool in 1987. **Robotic surgery** is a type of minimally invasive surgery (MIS). MIS differs from traditional surgery in that it is less invasive, meaning smaller incisions are made, which reduces the risk of infection; also, hospital stays are shorter, and recuperation time is reduced. Surgeons manipulate robotic arms to perform surgeries usually performed by humans. Although surgeons have to be trained in robotic surgery, use of a machine will reduce the effect of tremors in a surgeon's hands, which reduces any errors.

As robotic surgery became more popular, the National Aeronautics and Space Administration (NASA) developed the concept of **telesurgery**, which combines virtual reality, robots, and medicine. The U.S. Army also became involved in robotic surgery because it was interested in bringing surgery to soldiers who were on the battlefield and needed surgery immediately. The U.S. Army hoped robotic surgery would reduce war mortality rates (Robotic Surgery, 2012). Studies have indicated that some procedures such as an appendectomy demonstrate very little difference in outcome whether performed via the traditional method or the robotic method. However, robotic surgeries performed on the prostate have shown positive significant outcomes (The Next Generation, 2012). The robotic system that has dominated the current market is the **da Vinci Surgical System**, which was developed by Intuitive Surgical of Sunnyvale, California. It is used in cardiac, urologic, gynecologic, and general surgery. This tool was used in only 1,500 cases in 2000, which increased to 48,000 cases in 2006. The initial investment for a da Vinci Surgical System is $1.75 million, with an annual upkeep of $100,000. It has been approved by the Food and Drug Administration for several types of surgery (daVinci.Surgery, 2012). Despite the initial cost, experts feel that the actual procedure is cost effective because recuperation time is reduced for patients. Medical students will also have an opportunity to be trained in a robotic surgery fellowship once their initial education has been completed. Indications are that robotic surgery will continue to evolve as a surgical tool. As with any technological advances, the costs should decrease over time, and the tool will become more advanced and more efficient.

HRM Training in Technology

As the healthcare industry continues to use IT in its clinical and organization operations, and as IT departments, management, and HR departments continue to provide training for healthcare employees, the employees must be cognizant of the impact IT has on patients. Patients also require orientation to any IT care, and senior management must recognize the importance of IT to the success of its healthcare organization. According to Bernstein, McCreless, and Cote (2007), there are two conditions that are needed for success in IT integration in health care: a sufficient budget for IT upgrades to ensure it can support any needed clinical innovations, and recognition by senior leadership of the importance of IT in organization operations.

Role of the Chief Information Officer in Technology

As more healthcare services are delivered electronically, healthcare organizations have designated a **chief information officer** (CIO) to manage the organization's information systems. Some organizations may refer to this position as **chief technology officer** (CTO) or they may have both positions. Normally, the CIO is a vice president of the organization, and the CTO reports to that position. The CIO also integrates HIT into the organization's strategic plan. The CIO must have knowledge of current information technologies as they apply to the healthcare industry and of how new technology can apply to the organization. The CIO is also responsible for motivating employees whenever there is any technological change (Oz, 2006). C. Martin Harris, CIO of the Cleveland Clinic, believes that the challenge of the CIO is to move from implementing the EHR to continuing to provide quality patient care by developing an integrated system model. As more healthcare is being delivered by technology, it will be the responsibility of the CIO to develop a model that is patient oriented rather than operations oriented (Harris, 2008).

■ Teamwork in Health Care

The IOM report *To Err Is Human: Building a Safer Health System* describes the issues of preventable medical errors, which, according to the report, are in part the result of poor teamwork implementation. The report further states that effective teamwork can increase effective patient care. The report recommends that a team-training performance curriculum model should be developed that can be used in healthcare settings.

According to Lerner, Magrane, and Friedman (2009), there has been insufficient direction about how team training should be implemented. Healthcare teams can focus on quality improvement, delivery, and overall management. Both quality improvement and management teams are charged with improving organizational quality. These teams can be focused on one area of the organization or on the entire organization. Objectives are established to improve quality performance in designated areas. **Care delivery teams** are based on the type of population such as geriatrics or diabetics or on care settings such as an emergency room. Team protocols are developed based on the type of population. Simulations are a common practice in team training. Developed in 1987, the **Anesthesia Crisis Resource Management program** is one of the best team-training simulation programs. In this simulation, anesthesiologists manage a simulated patient during a surgical procedure in which medical crises are triggered so that the trainees can practice crisis management (Gaba, Howard, Fish, Smith & Sowb, 2001).

Rather than providing team training in the work environment, there have been suggestions that team training should be provided during medical education. Developed in the 1950s by medical faculty at Case Western University School of Medicine, **problem-based learning** consists of a structured education activity, performed in a small-group format, which uses case study analysis to solve medical problems in a collaborative setting. These are medical problems that medical students are likely to encounter during their professional careers. Larry Michaelson developed **team-based learning,** which is a tool that can be used for healthcare provider education. The instructor teaches several small groups in one classroom. Members take an examination independently and then as a group retake the examination to develop consensual answers. Each group shares its answers. Both the groups and the individuals are assessed on their performance (Lerner, Magrane & Friedman, 2009).

TeamSTEPPS

A recent government initiative that is team based is the U.S. Department of Defense and Agency for Healthcare Research and Quality collaborative effort resulting in Team Strategies and Tools to Enhance Patient Safety (**TeamSTEPPS**). This program promotes patient safety through team leadership, situational analysis, monitoring, collaboration, and communication. Communication is key in this program. It allows the opportunity for all involved, including the patient, to clarify any issues. There are three phases to this program: (1) assessment, (2) planning, training, and implementation, and (3) sustainment. The Agency for Healthcare Research and Quality and the U.S. Department of Defense have joined forces with the American Institutes for Research to develop a national implementation of this program. The purpose of this training is to develop master trainers who can train healthcare employees nationally in teamwork principles (About TeamSTEPPS, 2011).

Interprofessional Education

A form of teamwork is **interprofessional education** (IPE), which occurs when two or more professionals from different healthcare sectors engage in a dialogue so they can learn from each other—promoting interprofessional interaction. IPE promotes effective collaboration during patient care. It is an effective way of providing different perspectives of how to care for a patient within a team. According to Reeves, Goldman, and Oandasan (2007), an interprofessional interaction should have a balance of different healthcare professions and 5 to 10 members, with an expert facilitator playing a pivotal role in the learning process. IPE should provide learner-focused, faculty-focused, and organization-focused activities. Learner-focused activities include interactive learning such as problem-based activities with a clear clinical focus. The faculty-focused component should include a faculty training tool. The training should be organizationally focused to ensure that it is appropriate for the type of facility. The trainees must recognize the relevance of the training to their daily responsibilities.

Accountable Care Organization

Another form of teamwork in health care is the **accountable care organization** (ACO), which consists of a network of organizations and healthcare providers that offers coordinated care. ACOs coordinate both clinical and fiscal services. They are accountable to improve clinical outcomes for designated populations. If the outcomes are met or exceeded, the group of physicians receives a financial bonus. There may be excessive penalties for not reaching the targets (Gold, 2011). The model's assumption is that a provider team achieves or exceeds its stated objectives because of peer pressure. Services offered by an ACO can be a coordination of services offered by a tertiary hospital, home healthcare and hospice, rehabilitation, financing, education, social services, and preventive care. For example, a hospital may integrate physician practices as part of its system. The purpose of an ACO is to reduce costs and improve patient services (Integrated Delivery Systems Governing Board Manual, 2011).

This is not a new concept: It was introduced in the 1930s but became more popular in the 1980s and 1990s. However, with the downturn in the economy and the continued outcries for reform, the concept of an ACO has become more popular. There are approximately 100 U.S. ACOs with an estimated 40 million enrolled in this type of structure. Mayo, Kaiser Permanente, Harvard Pilgrim Health Care, and Intermountain have developed successful ACO models (Enthoven, 2009). The disadvantages of these types of systems are the onerous reporting and excessive penalties if the target outcomes are not achieved, which are major drawbacks. As healthcare costs continue to increase, the ACOs may be a viable option, but more ACOs need to be implemented nationally to determine their effectiveness.

A type of ACO model is **pay for performance** (P4P) or **value-based purchasing** (VBP), which are terms that describe healthcare payment systems that reward healthcare providers for their efficiency, which is defined as providing higher quality care for less cost. From a healthcare consumer perspective, the stakeholders should hold healthcare providers accountable for both the cost and high quality of their care. Because most health care in the United States has been historically provided by employers, in VBP, employers select healthcare plans based on demonstrated performance of quality and cost-effective health care (Theory and Reality of Value Based Purchasing, 2012). For the past decade, the Centers for Medicare and Medicaid Services has been collaborating with the National Quality Forum, the Joint Commission, the National Committee for Quality Assurance, the Agency for Healthcare Research and Quality, and the American Medical Association to implement initiatives to assess P4P systems nationwide. Despite national recommendations and successful programs that have been implemented nationwide, these efforts remain experimental because of lack of empirical evidence (Damburg, Raube, Teleki & dela Cruz, 2009).

For example, California's **Integrated Health Care Association** (IHA) operates the largest experimental P4P program nationally. The program, which began in 2003, targets 225 medical groups (representing 35,000 physicians) that contracted with the seven largest health maintenance organizations and point-of-service plans in the state, and it has 6.2 million enrollees. The IHA scored physician care based on the Healthcare Effectiveness Data and Information Set (HEDIS) measure and made performance-based payments. Results indicated that 25 of the physician organizations believed that the P4P positively affected behavior by focusing on quality accountability, 21 physician groups hired more staff to capture data to demonstrate their results, and 29 of the groups modified incentives to increase physician quality activities (Damberg, Raube, Teleki & dela Cruz, 2009). However, despite these positive results, there were no major breakthrough improvements in quality. Questions regarding the amount and type of incentives need to be reevaluated. In addition, the type of quality indicators may also need to be reevaluated. P4P is a valid concept for health care. As programs that are more experimental are evaluated, lessons that were learned from the first round of experimental programs must be taken into account. Despite these efforts, employers seldom use this type of information when selecting benefits for their workers. A recent telephone interview of 609 employers in 41 markets, which represented 78% of the urban U.S. population, indicated that premium rates and geographic coverage motivated their decisions. Despite these issues, the Futurescan: Healthcare Trends and Implications 2006–2011 survey indicates that P4P will become more commonplace (Rosenthal et al., 2007).

From a strategic standpoint, if a hospital decides to integrate other services into its operations, the first step is to assess what services are needed for continuum of care in the geographic area. This initiative should also be consistent with the mission, vision statement, and strategy of the organization.

■ Nursing Home Trends

In 2001, the Robert Wood Johnson Foundation funded a pilot project developed by Dr. Bill Thomas, the **Green House Project**, which is a unique type of nursing home established as a residence that provides services—that is, a home to the residents rather than an institution at which to receive care. The concept alters the size of the facility, the physical environment, and the delivery of services (Fine, 2009). The home is managed by a team of workers who share the care of the residents, including the cooking and housekeeping. The daily staff members are certified nursing assistants. All mandated professional personnel such as physicians, nurses, social workers, and dieticians form visiting clinical support teams that assess the elders and supervise their care (Kane, Lum, Cutler, Degenholtz & Yu, 2007).

The residents can eat their meals when they choose. The word "patient" is not used—all residents are called "elders." The Green House is designed for 6 to 10 elders. Each resident has a private room and private bathroom. The elder rooms have high levels of sunlight and are located near the kitchen and dining area. There are patios and gardens for elders and staff to enjoy. Although these new types of nursing homes look like a residential home, they adhere to all long-term housing requirements. A Green House looks like other homes in its designated neighborhood (Fine, 2009).

Residents can have their own pets, which are not allowed in traditional nursing homes. According to a recent study performed by the University of Minnesota, the residents of the Green House are able to perform their activities of daily living longer and are less depressed than residents of traditional nursing homes and are able to be self-sufficient longer than residents of traditional nursing homes. The staff also enjoys working at the Green House, and there is less staff turnover (Kane et al., 2007).

The first Green House was constructed in Tupelo, Mississippi. There are now 18 Green Houses nationwide. Dr. Thomas eventually partnered with NCB Capital Impact, which is a not-for-profit organization that provides financial assistance to underserved communities. NCB Capital Impact has a loan program that provides financial assistance up to $125,000 to support engineering and architectural and other expenses for a selected Green House site. The borrower must contribute 25% of the loan amount (The Green House Project, 2012). There are currently 18 Green Houses across the United States.

■ Social Media Communication

There are several definitions of **social media,** but the prevailing concept of the definitions is that social media has an electronic platform and it is used as a tool for interaction between individuals or organizations. It can be used as a communication tool and as a marketing tool. Social media is being used by healthcare organizations as a recruiting tool. Social media has also become a communication tool for patient engagement and for employees and providers. According to a September 2011 employee survey of IT professionals, administrators, and physicians, 75% use social media for professional purposes within their employment. The Mayo Clinic and the U.S. Department of Veterans Affairs are exploring ways to use social media for patient engagement including education (Most Health IT Pros Use Social Media, 2011).

Hospitals and academic medical centers are establishing more YouTube channels and Twitter accounts nationwide. Physicians use Twitter to communicate easily and quickly with other physicians. YouTube provides an opportunity for brief healthcare education videos.

Social media can be easily used as part of a health communications program. Because of the continued increase in social media use, the Centers for Disease Control and Prevention Health Communicator's Social Media Toolkit (2010) contains recommendations for social media use in the healthcare industry:

1. Perform market research to determine key educational messages.
2. Review social media sites by user statistics and demographics.
3. Start a social media campaign by using low-risk tools such as podcasts and videos.
4. The educational messages must be based in science.
5. Develop a system of easy viral sharing by patients so everyone can benefit from the message.
6. Social media users should listen to each other. If patients are voicing concerns or questions, they need to be answered.
7. Leverage social networks to expand the message. An average Facebook user has 130 friends that they can easily share a health message with.

In addition to these recommendations, the federal government has established two websites for social media best practices and governance policies: http://govsocmed.pbworks.com/Web-2-0-Governance-Policies-and-Best-Practices and http://socialmediagovernance.com/policies.php.

As with any trend, it is the responsibility of the organization to offer training in these types of tools to ensure responsible use. The HR department would collaborate with senior management and the IT department to ensure that these IT tools are used appropriately.

■ Conclusion

Healthcare trends have been impacted by two major factors: technology and consumer preferences. Each factor has impacted on how healthcare delivery services are provided. This chapter discussed different technological trends and consumer preferences in healthcare. HR must provide ongoing training and development to their employees to ensure they are current with any new trends. Like other industries, healthcare organizations must maintain a competitive advantage by providing quality and innovative health care that satisfies their healthcare customer.

■ Vocabulary

Accountable care organization
American Health Information
   Community
Anesthesia Crisis Resource
   Management Program
Care delivery teams
Chief information officer
Chief technology officer
Cleveland Clinic
Cultural competency
Culturally competent healthcare
   organization
da Vinci Surgical System
Duke University Health Systems
Electronic health record
Electronic medical record
E-prescribing
Globalization of health care
Green House Project
Health Information Technology for
   Economic and Clinical Health Act
   of 2009
Host country nationals
Integrated Health Care Association

Interprofessional education
Joint Commission
Meaningful use
Medical tourism
National Alliance for Health
   Information Technology
National Committee on Quality
   Assurance
National eHealth Collaborative
National Healthcare Disparities
   Report
Office of the National Coordinator
   for Information Technology
Pay for performance
Problem-based learning
Robotic surgery
Social media
Strategic cultural plan
Team-based learning
TeamSTEPPS
Telemedicine
Telesurgery
Value-based purchasing
Workplace diversity

■ References

About TeamSTEPPS (2011). Available at: http://teamstepps.ahrq.gov/about-2cl_3.htm. Accessed April 23, 2011.

About Medical Tourism (2012). Available at: http://www.medicaltourismassociation.com/Accreditation.jsp. Accessed March 12, 2012.

Anderson, R., Rice, T. & Kominski, G. (2007). *Changing the U.S. Health Care System*. San Francisco, CA: Jossey-Bass.

Andrulis, D. (2003). Reducing racial and ethnic disparities in disease management to improve health outcomes. *Practical Disease Management*, 11(12):789–800.

Bernstein, M., McCreless, T. & Cote, M. (2007). Five constants of information of technology in healthcare. *Hospital Topics*, 85(1):17–25.

Betancourt, J., Green, A. & Carrillo, J. (2002). *Cultural Competencies in Health Care: Emerging Frameworks and Practical Approaches*. Available at: http://www.commonwealthfund.org/Publications/Fund-Reports/2002/Oct/Cultural-Competence-in-Health-Care--Emerging-Frameworks-and-Practical-Approaches.aspx. Accessed January 1, 2012.

Betancourt, J., Green, A., Carrillo, J. & Ananeh-Firempong II, O. (2003). Defining cultural competence: A practice framework for addressing racial/ethnic disparities in health and health care. *Public Health Reports*, 55(3):293–302.

Byars, L. & Rue, L. (2006). *Human Resource Management* (8th ed.). New York, NY: McGraw-Hill/Irwin, pp. 87–111.

Clark, P. (2009). Prejudice and the medical profession: A five year update. *Journal of Law, Medicine & Ethics*, 34(1):118–133.

Cleveland Clinic/Microsoft Pilot Promising: Home Health Services May Benefit Chronic Disease Management (2011). Available at: http://www.prnewswire.com/news-releases/cleveland-clinicmicrosoft-pilot-promising-home-health-services-may-benefit-chronic-disease-management-85811337.html. Accessed September 20, 2011.

Companion Global Healthcare, Inc. (2011). Available at: http://www.companionglobalhealthcare.com/about.aspx. Accessed April 23, 2011.

daVinci.Surgery (2012). Available at: http://www.davincisurgery.com/. Accessed January 20, 2012.

Damburg, C., Raube, K., Teleki, S. & dela Cruz, E. (2009). Taking stock of pay for performance: A candid assessment from the front lines. *Health Affairs*, 28(2):515–525.

Department of Health and Human Services (2011). Health information technology. Available at: http://www.hhs.gov/healthit/onc/background. Accessed May 21, 2011.

Diversity in the Workplace (2011). Available at: http://hr.fhda.edu/diversity/. Accessed September 15, 2011.

Ellis, B. & Shanley, C. (2011). The globalization of healthcare. Available at: http://www.hhmag.com/hhmag_app/jsp/articledisplay.jsp?dcrpath=HHNMAG. Accessed April 23, 2011.

Enthoven, A. (2009). Integrated delivery systems: The cure for fragmentation. *The Journal of Managed Care*, 15:S284–S290.

Fine, S. (2009). Where to live as we age. *Parade Magazine*, May 31: 8–9.

Gaba, D., Howard, S., Fish, K., Smith, B. & Sowb, Y. (2001). Simulation-based training in anesthesia crisis resource management (ACRM): A decade of experience. *Simulation & Gaming*, June: 175–191.

Gathers, D. (2003). Diversity management: An imperative for healthcare organizations. *Hospital Topics*, 81(3):14–19.

Gertner, E., Sabino, J., Mahady, E., Detrick, L., Patton, J., Grim, M., Geiger, J., Salas-Gold, J. (2011). Accountable care organizations, explained. Available at: http://www.npr.org/2011/04/01/132937232/accountable-care-organizations-explained. Accessed January 1, 2012.

Gold, J. (2011). *Accountable Care Organizations Explained*. Available at: http://www.npr.org/2011/04/01/132937232/accountable-care-organizations-explained. Accessed January 26, 2012.

Harris, C. M. (2008). C. Martin Harris, CIO, **Cleveland Clinic**. *Health Management Technology*, 29(7):10.

Health Communicator's Social Media Toolkit (2010). Available at: http://www.cdc.gov/healthcommunication/ToolsTemplates/SocialMediaToolkit_BM.pdf. Accessed September 18, 2011.

HealthVault (2012). Available at: http://www.healthvault.com/personal/websites-overview.html. Accessed January 1, 2012.

Hirsch, M. (2011). EHR safety: IOM report a good start, but more can be done. Available at: http://www.fierceemr.com/story/ehr-safety-ion-report-good-start-more-can-be-done/2011-1. Accessed January 1, 2012.

Horowitz, M., Rosensweig, J. & Jones, C. (2007). Medical tourism: Globalization of the healthcare marketplace. Available at: http://www.ncbi.nlm.nih.gov. Accessed April 10, 2011.

Hunt, B. (2007). Managing equality and cultural diversity in the health workforce. *Journal of Clinical Nursing*, 16:2252–2259.

Institute of Medicine (2001). *Crossing the Quality Chasm: A New Health System for the 21st Century*. Available at: http://www.iom.edu/Reports/2001/Crossing-the-Quality-Chasm-A-New-Health-System-for-the-21st-Century.aspx. Accessed July 15, 2011.

Integrated Delivery Systems Governing Board Manual (2011). Available at: http://www.whs-seattle.com/manual/integrateddelivery.html. Accessed September 14, 2011.

Kane, R., Lum, T., Cutler, L., Degenholtz, J. & Yu, T. (2007). Resident outcomes in small-house nursing homes. A longitudinal evaluation of the initial Green House program. *Journal of Geriatrics Society*, 55(6):832–839.

Lamont, J. (2010). Data drives decision making in healthcare. Available at: http://www.kmworld.com. Accessed April 23, 2011.

Landro, L. (2009). Incentives push more doctors to e-prescribe. Available at: http://www.online.wsj.com/article/SB12349533946000191.html. Accessed May 21, 2011.

Lerner, S., Magrane, D. & Friedman, E. (2009). Teaching teamwork in medical education. *Mount Sinai School of Medicine*, 76:318–329.

Medical Tourism: Statistics and Facts (2011). Available at: http://www.health-tourisim.com/medical-tourism/statistics. Accessed April 23, 2011.

Most Health IT Pros Use Social Media (2011). Available at: http://www.informationweek.com/news/healthcare/mobile-wireless/231601331. Accessed September 18, 2011.

National Alliance for Health Information Technology (2008). Available at: http://www.medicalnewstoday.com/articles/101878.php. Accessed May 21, 2011.

Next Generation (2012). Available at: http://www.nextgenmd.org/. Accessed January 20, 2012.

Oz, E. (2006). *Management Information Systems*. Mason, OH: Thomson South-Western.

Pavarini, P. (2009). The globalization of healthcare. Available at: http://www.szdhealthlawscan.com. Accessed April 10, 2011.

Reeves, S., Goldman, J., Oandasan, I. (2007). Key factors in planning and implementing interprofessional education in healthcare settings. *Journal of Allied Health*, 36(4):231–235.

Rosenthal, M., Landon, B., Normand, S., Frank, R., Ahmad, T. & Epstein, A. (2007). Employers' use of value-based purchasing strategies. *Journal of the American Medical Association*, 21:2281–2288.

Robotic Surgery (2012). Available at: http://biomed.brown.edu/Courses/BI108/BI108_2005_Groups/04/davinci.html. Accessed January 31, 2012.

Salisbury, J. & Byrd, S. (2006). Why diversity matters in healthcare. *CSA Bulletin*, Spring:90–94.

Shields, A., Shin, P., Leu, M., Levy, D., Betancourt, R., Hawkins, D., et al. (2007). Adoption of health information technology in community health centers: Results of a national survey. *Health Affairs*, 26(3):1373–1383.

Staff Qualifications (2011). Available at: http://my.clevelandclinic.org/abu-dhabi/careers/staff-qualifications.aspx. Accessed April 10, 2011.

Teich, J., Osheroff, J., Pifer, F., Sittig, D., Jenders, R. & CDS Expert Review Panel (2005). AMIA Position Paper: Clinical decision support in electronic prescribing: Recommendations and an action plan: Report of the Joint Clinical Decision Support Group. *Journal of the American Medical Informatics*, 12:365–378.

The Green House Project (2012). Available at: http://www.ncbcapitalimpact.org/default.aspx?id=146&terms=Green%20House. Accessed January 31, 2012.

Theory and Reality of Value Based Purchasing (2012). Available at: http://www.ahrq.gov/qual/meyerrpt. htm#head3. Accessed January 30. 2012.

Valerius, J. (2007). The electronic health record. What every information manager should know. *The Information Management Journal*, 4(1):56–59.

Ventres, W. & Shah, A. (2007). How do EHRs affect the physician-patient relationship? *American Family Physician*, 75(9):1385–1390.

Vreeman, D., Taggard, S., Rhine, M. & Worrell, T. (2006). Evidence for electronic health systems in physical therapy. *Physical Therapy*, 86(4):434–446.

What's Different About Rural Health Care? (2011). Available at: http://www.ruralhealthweb.org/go/ left/about-rural-health/what-s-different-about-rural-health-care. Accessed September 18, 2011.

Whitman, J. C. & David, S. (2007). Effectively integrating your EMR/HER initiative. *The Physician Executive*, 33(5):56–59.

Women in Healthcare Administration: Attaining Leadership Roles (2011). Available at: http://rndegrees .net/women-in-healthcare-administration.php. Accessed September 18, 2011.

STUDENT WORKBOOK ACTIVITY 10.1

Complete the following case scenarios based on the information provided in this chapter. You must use two vocabulary or key terms discussed in the text in each of your four answers. You can repeat two terms once.

Real-Life Applications: Case Scenario 1

Your healthcare organization has increased in diversity over the past 5 years, yet there has been no significant employee training to adapt to this new situation. Your manager has asked you to develop a proposal for employee training.

Activity

Define the concept of a culturally competent organization. Develop a training program that addresses the eight guidelines for cultural competency.

Responses

_____

_____

_____

_____

_____

Real-Life Applications: Case Scenario 2

You realize your father, who is underinsured, cannot afford the copayment for his liver transplant. He has asked your advice on what to do next.

Activity

Explain the concept of medical tourism to him and provide statistical information regarding which countries offer different types of medical services.

_____

_____

_____

_____

_____

Real-Life Applications: Case Scenario 3

Your hospital has decided to develop a strategic alliance with a healthcare organization in China and has asked you to work in China for 12 months during the transition period for the employees who will be working there.

Activity

Discuss the differences in international management that must be addressed.

Responses

_____

_____

_____

_____

_____

Real-Life Applications: Case Scenario 4

As the office manager of a physician practice that sees primarily Medicare patients, you have been asked by one of the physicians to research EHRs and e-prescribing. She has heard the federal government is giving bonuses for technology use.

Activity

Research information on the EHR, and provide three advantages and three disadvantages of using an EHR. Discuss the concept of meaningful use to your boss.

Responses

_____

_____

_____

_____

STUDENT WORKBOOK ACTIVITY 10.2

In Your Own Words

Please describe these core concepts in your own words.

Cultural competency:

_____

_____

_____

_____

Medical tourism:

_____

_____

_____

_____

Culturally competent organization:

_____

_____

_____

_____

Telemedicine:

_____

_____

_____

_____

Team-based learning:

_____

_____

_____

_____

Problem-based learning:

_____

_____

_____

_____

Strategic cultural plan:

_____

_____

_____

_____

Host country national:

_____

_____

_____

_____

Meaningful use:

_____

_____

_____

_____

Electronic health record:

_____

_____

_____

_____

STUDENT WORKBOOK ACTIVITY 10.3

Internet Exercises

Write your answers in the spaces provided.

- Visit each of the websites that are listed in the text that follows.
- Name the organization.
- Locate its mission statement on its website. If the organization does not have a mission statement, describe its purpose.
- Provide a brief overview of the activities of the organization.
- Apply this organization to the chapter information.

Websites
http://www.companionglobalhealthcare.com

Organization name:

_____

Mission statement:

_____

_____

_____

Overview of activities:

_____

_____

_____

Application to chapter information:

_____

_____

_____

http://www.health-tourism.com

Organization name:

_____

Mission statement:

_____

_____

_____

Overview of activities:

_____

_____

_____

Application to chapter information:

_____

_____

_____

http://www.diversityconnection.org

Organization name:

_____

Mission statement:

_____

_____

Overview of activities:

_____

_____

_____

Application to chapter information:

_____

_____

_____

http://teamstepps.ahrq.gov
Organization name:

_____

Mission statement:

_____

_____

_____

Overview of activities:

_____

_____

_____

Application to chapter information:

_____

_____

_____

http://www.medicaltourismassociation.com

Organization name:

_____

Mission statement:

_____

_____

_____

Overview of activities:

_____

_____

_____

Application to chapter information:

_____

_____

_____

http://www.hhs.gov/healthit/

Organization name:

_____

Mission statement:

_____

_____

_____

Overview of activities:

_____

_____

_____

Application to chapter information:

_____

_____

_____

STUDENT ACTIVITY 10.4: DISCUSSION BOARDS FOR ONLINE, HYBRID, AND TRADITIONAL ONGROUND CLASSES

Discussion Board Guidelines

The discussion board is used in online and web-enhanced courses in place of classroom lectures and discussion. The board can be an enhancement to traditional classes. The discussion board is the way in which the students "link together" as a class. The following are guidelines to help focus on the discussion topic and to define the roles and responsibilities of the discussion coordinator and other members of the class. The educator will be the discussion moderator for this course.

1. The educator will post the discussion topic and directions for the upcoming week. These postings should all be responses to the original topic or responses to other students' responses. When people respond to what someone else has posted, they should start the posting with the person's name so it is clear which

message they are responding to. **A response such as "Yes" or "I agree" does not count for credit. Your responses must be in your own words. You cannot copy and paste from the text.**

2. Postings (especially responses) should include enough information so the message is clear but should not be so long that it becomes difficult to follow. Remember, this is like talking to someone in a classroom setting. The postings should reflect the content of the text or other assignments. If you retrieve information from the Internet, the hyperlink must be cited.

3. Students should check the discussion daily to see if new information has been posted that requires their attention and response.

Good discussion will often include different points of view. Students should feel free to disagree or "challenge" others to support their positions or ideas. All discussions must be handled in a respectful manner. The following are discussion boards for this chapter.

Discussion Boards

1. Health care is now a global industry. Support or refuse this statement. Be specific.
2. Why do you think medical tourism has developed? Would you participate in it? Why or why not?
3. EHR systems are being implemented across the United States. What are the positives and negatives of this trend? What is meaningful use?
4. Discuss the different ways employees can be trained in teamwork in health care. Do you like working in teams? Why or why not?

Strategic Human Resource Management

Learning Objectives

The student will be able to:

- Define strategy.
- Prepare a Porter's Five Forces analysis.
- Differentiate between a mission statement and a vision statement.
- Prepare a strengths, weaknesses, opportunities, and threats analysis.
- Evaluate the macroenvironmental forces in the healthcare industry.
- Discuss the importance of workforce planning.

DID YOU KNOW THAT?

- A mission statement is the foundation for a realistic and achievable organizational goal.
- The Institute of Medicine defines *quality* in health care as patient services current with scientific knowledge that result in a desired health outcome.
- Workforce planning is a biannual or annual method of determining future job openings.
- A succession plan identifies replacements for key organizational positions.
- A labor budget projects staffing levels, overtime costs, employee benefits, payroll, unemployment taxes, and any financial incentives.

■ Introduction: Quality and Strategy Concepts

Organizational Quality

A strategic goal of any healthcare organization is the quality performance of the employees. The Institute of Medicine (1998) created the most accepted definition of

quality in the healthcare industry: patient services current with scientific knowledge that result in a desired health outcome. This definition targets the relationship between the provider and the patient or population. In addition to this relationship are the additional activities and the structure involved in the provision of care. This would include the facility itself and other personnel directly or indirectly involved in patient care. To maintain a high-quality organization, the human resources (HR) department provides policies and procedures for all organizational levels. This concept of quality is inherent in healthcare strategic planning to ensure that quality is a long-term strategic objective.

Strategic Concepts

A **strategy** is management's plan for operating the organization over the long term. Management typically is committed to a set of long-term actions to operate an organization. The goal of a strategy is to achieve a competitive advantage. The process of crafting a strategy consists of:

1. Mission and vision statements.
2. Performance objectives.
3. A strategy to achieve the objectives.
4. Strategy execution.
5. Performance evaluations and development of corrective actions based on the evaluations (Thompson, Strickland & Gamble, 2010).

A mission statement describes an organization's current activities and purpose. A vision statement provides guidance about the aspirations of an organization. With any mission and vision statements, the role of the HR department is to ensure there are employees in place that have the skills and knowledge to achieve the mission and vision of the organization.

Financial and strategic objectives measure the performance of an organization to ensure the organization is achieving its mission and working toward its vision. HR can contribute to performance measurement by developing **human capital metrics**. Once the objectives are developed, a strategy is developed and executed based on the capabilities of the organization and the influences of the external environment. A strengths, weaknesses, opportunities, and threats (SWOT) analysis is performed prior to strategy development. In addition to an SWOT analysis, a Porter's Five Forces analysis is performed to assess the industry's conditions to determine what strategy can be implemented to give an organization a competitive advantage. The Five Forces analysis examines forces in an industry: barriers to entry, competition, buyers, suppliers, and substitute products or services that are available to buyers. Once the strategy is executed, an evaluation of the company performance to assess its success is performed. A strategy may be changed based on the evaluation process.

Recruiting, training, developing, and retaining appropriate employees is a fundamental human resource management (HRM) process that contributes to the strategic planning process because the appropriate human capital is needed to achieve both short-term and long-term success. The HR department should align its policies with the strategic planning of the organization to ensure a sustained competitive advantage. The HR department can also contribute to the success of **strategic management** by developing metrics to assess human capital performance (Inyang, 2010). This chapter will focus on the five steps of strategy development and implementation introduced earlier in this section and the role of HRM in the strategic management process.

■ Development of Mission and Vision Statements

Graham and Havlick (1994) state that a strong **mission statement** should include four elements: the purpose, the specific business, geographic location, and customer base. According to Hader (2006), a mission statement should be more than just a written exercise. It should be the foundation of a realistic and attainable goal. To develop a mission statement appropriate for the organization, senior management should ask for initial input from employees, review organizational documents, and, as the mission evolves, involve continued input from employees at all levels. An active agenda should be developed to educate staff on how to achieve the mission of the organization. In addition, there should be an evaluation process of activities of the organization to ensure that the mission statement is achieved by all employees. Table 11.1 lists examples of healthcare mission statements. Some organizations have only a one-sentence mission statement, and other organizations have a mission statement that comprises several sentences.

Once a mission statement is developed, a vision statement will also be crafted for the organization. Whereas a **mission statement** focuses on current operations, the **vision statement** focuses on where the organization is headed. It is a futuristic statement. It contains a long-term goal and often includes information about how the organization is going to achieve the goal. It often is an inspiring statement of the organization's ultimate goal. Table 11.1 lists examples of healthcare mission statements from two federal government organizations—the Federal Emergency Management Agency and the Centers for Disease Control and Prevention—and one from the world-renowned healthcare organization, the Mayo Clinic. Each of these organizations have developed one powerful statement that clearly indicates the overall focus of their organizations. These statements reveal to both their employees and the world their organizational priority.

Once a mission statement is developed, a vision statement will also be crafted for the organization. Whereas a mission statement focuses on current operations, the vision

Table 11.1 Healthcare Organizations' Mission Statements

Federal Emergency Management Agency

FEMA's mission is to support our citizens and first responders to ensure that as a nation we work together to build, sustain, and improve our capability to prepare for, protect against, respond to, recover from, and mitigate all hazards.

Centers for Disease Control and Prevention

Collaborating to create the expertise, information, and tools that people and communities need to protect their health—through health promotion, prevention of disease, injury and disability, and preparedness for new health threats.

Mayo Clinic

The Mayo Clinic will provide the best care to every patient, every day, through integrated clinical practice, education, and research.

Source: Federal Emergency Management Agency (2011), Centers for Disease Control and Prevention (2011), and Courtesy of the Mayo Foundation for Medical Education and Research.

statement focuses on where the organization is headed. It is a futuristic statement. It contains a long-term goal and often includes information about how the organization is going to achieve the goal. It often is an inspiring statement of the organization's ultimate goal.

Table 11.2 contains three vision statements of different healthcare organizations: Resurrection Health Care, a Chicago-based Catholic healthcare organization; a global pharmaceutical company, Pfizer, Inc.; and the world-renowned healthcare organization, the Dana-Farber Cancer Institute. Although the mission statement is important because it provides a framework for current operations of the organization, the vision statement is equally important because it tells everyone what is important to the organization over the long term. The Resurrection Health Care vision statement reflects the organization's focus on expanding its Chicago base and becoming a national leader in healthcare delivery. Pfizer's vision is to develop new drugs to eradicate diseases. The Dana-Farber Cancer Institute's vision is to eradicate cancer and other major chronic diseases. Like the mission statements, these vision statements are formulated to inspire employees and the world about the future plans of their organization.

Once mission and vision statements are formulated, a separate mission and vision statement should be formulated by each department of the organization. The departments of each organization must develop a mission and vision statement that complements the corporate mission and vision statement. These lower-level statements will further strengthen the focus of the organization.

Table 11.2 Healthcare Organizations' Vision Statements

Resurrection Health Care

Resurrection Health Care, the leading Catholic health care system in Chicagoland, will transform into a patient-centered integrated regional health system that is recognized as a national leader in delivering quality outcomes to the patients and communities it serves.

Pfizer Inc.

At Pfizer, we're inspired by a single goal: your health. That's why we're dedicated to developing new, safe medicines to prevent and treat the world's most serious diseases. And why we are making them available to the people who need them most. We believe that from progress comes hope and the promise of a healthier world.

Dana-Farber Cancer Institute

Dana-Farber Cancer Institute's ultimate goal is the eradication of cancer, AIDS, and related diseases and the fear that they engender.

Courtesy of Resurrection Health Care Corporation, the Dana-Farber Cancer Institute, and Pfizer Inc.

■ Development of Performance Objectives

Once the mission and vision statements are created, objectives are developed, which are quantifiable target statements to measure the performance of an organization. Objectives should be quantifiable and have a deadline for achievement. Typically, there are two types of objectives: financial and strategic. **Financial objectives** are lagging indicators of an organization's performance. They measure what the organization has already accomplished. **Strategic objectives** are leading indicators of what the organization would like to achieve. Strategic objectives focus on market standing and improving competitive vitality (Thompson, Peteraf, Gamble & Strickland, 2012). Examples of financial objectives are (1) increase annual revenues by 18% or (2) increase annual profit margins by 3%. Financial objectives measure what the organization's performance was in the past. Historical financial data are analyzed to assess if the objective was achieved. Examples of strategic objectives are (1) increase market presence 10% by 2013 and (2) acquire one healthcare agency by 2015. Strategic objectives measure what future action will be taken by the organization.

This type of objective setting is a **balanced scorecard approach**. Developed by Kaplan and Norton in the 1990s, the balanced approach is used to assess an organization's performance by setting both financial and performance objectives. Financial data as well as business operations, customer management, and HR

Table 11.3 The Duke Balanced Scorecard

Clinical Quality & Internal Business	Customer Service
Goal: Faster enhanced clinical care and new program development to improve quality, patient safety, and efficiency.	Goal: Continuously improve customer service for both internal and external customers.
Work Culture	**Finances**
Goal: Continuously improve the work culture consistent with the DUHS value proposition.	Goal: Generate sufficient resources to reinvest in people, technology, buildings, research, and education.

Source: Duke Human Resources (2011).

data are collected to provide a balanced view of performance (Balanced Scorecard Basics, 2011).

The balanced scorecard approach is becoming more common in the healthcare industry. Duke University Health System uses this approach. Table 11.3 outlines the Duke Balanced Scorecard. The Duke University Health System (DUHS) HR department assesses the performance of employees by evaluating them in the following key areas: customer service, finances, work culture, and clinical quality and internal business. If DUHS focuses on improving work culture and customer service, the clinical quality and financial objectives will improve also. Based on these four quadrants, employees are assessed on their behavior and their expected job result, their adherence to the DUHS cultural norms, and whether they have achieved goals in each of the quadrants. These quadrants are tied to the mission of DUHS. DUHS has an overall goal for each quadrant. Each department and individual employee would have a goal tied to the DUHS goal. For example, the DUHS goal of clinical quality and internal business is to foster enhanced clinical care and new program development for patient safety and efficiency. The personal goal of a DUHS nurse would be to demonstrate the provision of quality patient care. This nurse's department goal would be the implementation of 100% error-free patient care for 6 months. By using the balanced scorecard approach, DUHS believes it will continue to be a high-performance organization (Duke Human Resources, 2011). That is the power of the balanced scorecard. Once these internal goals are developed, the next step is to assess the external environment of the organization.

■ Macroenvironment Analysis

A **macroenvironment** analysis is influenced by two levels of the external environment: the macroenvironment and the immediate or industry environment. The macroenvironment is composed of the following influences: economic, technologic, sociocultural, demographic, governmental, and legal (Thompson et al., 2012). Each of these influences can impact a healthcare organization. As an example, consider the macroenvironmental influences on a hospital's decision to expand its facility to increase potential revenues. The hospital's options are to operate an elective surgery center or to start a home healthcare agency.

Economic Influences

Economic influences can occur at the national and local levels. During the past 3 to 5 years, the United States has experienced an economic downturn, resulting in a 10% unemployment rate (U.S. Unemployment Rate, 2011). Those unemployed individuals who lost their employee healthcare insurance would replace their health care by visiting a hospital emergency room or an emergency care facility, thereby placing more stress on these components of the healthcare system. These economic conditions may or may not be occurring at the local level, but most likely there will be an impact because of national conditions. Elective surgery would not be an option during difficult economic times because it is not a need. At this stage of analysis, elective surgery is eliminated from the expansion options for the hospital, and it appears that a home health agency is the choice.

Governmental and Legal Influences

The healthcare industry is one of the most heavily regulated industries in the United States, so federal, state, and local regulations for a health agency are examined. In addition, communication with different accrediting bodies for each option would also be necessary to assess accreditation costs. If the facility will serve both Medicare and Medicaid patients, there will be regulations from these agencies. A cost–benefit analysis will be performed to assess the cost of adhering to these regulations.

Technologic Influences

Advances in technology have led to new capabilities in patient care through improved medical procedures and equipment. Technologic advances in portable medical equipment have increased the number of home healthcare agencies. More care can be provided on an outpatient basis because of these advances. Another major technologic advance is the development of the electronic medical record, which allows rapid transfer of patient information electronically. This could have a positive impact on home health care, increasing the efficiency of its operations.

Sociocultural Influences

Sociocultural influences are consumer preferences based on lifestyles and values. They directly influence major decisions. This is the most important macroenvironmental factor in determining a strategy. Consumer preferences dictate profits. Research indicates that consumers prefer home health care during a prolonged illness rather than a hospital stay. In a recent survey of 1,000 U.S. adults, more than 80% preferred home health care (Tellez, 2011). More insurance plans, both private and public, are reimbursing home health agency care because the care is cost effective.

Demographic Influences

Demographic influences include age, race, income levels, ethnicity, geographic location, education, family size, and life expectancies. Statistics indicate the population is living and working longer, which results in chronic healthcare conditions. Therefore, development of a home healthcare agency may be an option for the hospital for these reasons. The impact of the Patient Protection and Affordability Care Act of 2010, which focuses on cost containment, may also be a reason for implementing a home health agency.

Before making a final decision on this option, the second portion of the environmental analysis is the industry analysis. Michael E. Porter (1979) developed the concept of a Five Forces analysis, which outlines the five forces that impact industry success: competition, suppliers, substitute products, new entrants into the industry, and buyers.

■ Industry Environment, or Porter's Five Forces Analysis

According to Michael E. Porter, the **attractiveness of an industry**, or how profitable an industry can be for a company, is the result of five competitive pressures in the market: rivalry or competition, suppliers of resources needed by the organization, substitute products or alternative services that a customer can choose, potential new organizations entering the industry, and buyers of the product or service. According to Porter, each force needs to be assessed by its level of power over the organization—low power, medium power, or high power of influencing the organization's efforts to be profitable. If the analysis indicates these forces have high power, then it may be a poor decision to open a home health agency. If it is determined that the forces have low power, then this may be an opportunity for the hospital to increase revenues (Porter, 1979). The following is an analysis of the hospital's industry using **Porter's Five Forces model** to assess whether opening a home health agency is a viable option.

Rivalry/Competition Forces

Competition is the strongest force of the five forces. If there are several home healthcare agencies that would compete directly with the hospital's new agency, then it may not be the best opportunity for the hospital to increase its revenues. Existing agencies may already have a dominant market share. The hospital may still have an opportunity to start a home health agency, but it may determine that it should be placed in a different geographic location. If it is determined that there are existing home health agencies that have dominated the market, then the power of the competition is high. If there are few competitors in this market, then the power of the competition is low, and therefore the opportunity is more attractive. *Analysis: low to high power.*

Suppliers Force

Suppliers provide materials or labor for an organization. The more specialized and unique a product or service is, the more power the supplier will have over an organization. In this instance, the suppliers for a home health agency would consist of the medical personnel and medical equipment. Medical equipment could be obtained from different suppliers; therefore the power the supplier would have over the organization would *most likely be low*. Depending on the types of services offered, *supplier power could be low to high*. Many home health agencies offer general assistance to homebound individuals, so these employees would be easy to hire. With continued nursing labor shortages, supplier power could be medium to high. *Analysis: low to high power.*

Substitute Products Force

Substitute products or services are any alternatives a consumer would have to select instead of a home healthcare agency service. A substitute product or service could be a family member caring for the individual. Another option could be placing the homebound individual in an institution. Both are options but have limitations. A family member often becomes exhausted from this type of care and eventually opts for home health care. Using an institution for health care may be expensive and require additional copayments from the family or individual. *Analysis: low to medium power.*

Barriers to Entry Force

Barriers to entry refers to the limitations that are imposed on a potential competitor to entering the home healthcare industry. Barriers to entry typically include high capital requirements, high level of regulation, specialized knowledge needed to enter the industry, or the power of existing competition already present in the market. Start-up costs for a home health agency are not high. There could be some issues with labor supply shortages, which could be one barrier. If there are many government regulations that an organization must adhere to, these would be a barrier to entry. *Analysis: low to medium power.*

Consumers/Buyers Force

Buyer forces' power is linked to how many substitute products there are, how frequently the buyer purchases the service, how loyal the buyer is to an existing provider, and if there is a cost for a buyer to switch to another service provider. There would not be any costs involved in switching from one home health agency to another, provided the insurance covers the new agency. The main reason that consumer power would be high is because most consumers have strong loyalty to their healthcare providers and often form bonds with them. A well-developed marketing strategy would need to be developed to emphasize superior customer care. *Analysis: high power.*

The Porter's Five Forces analysis indicates there is a mix of low to high power of the five forces. If the new agency is structured appropriately, the power of the five forces could be limited to low. Potentially, this industry could be attractive. However, to assess the success of this industry choice, a SWOT analysis must be performed in conjunction with Porter's Five Forces analysis.

■ SWOT Analysis

A **SWOT** analysis examines the strengths and weaknesses of a company and the opportunities of a company (what situations are available to the company that could be positive for their position), as well as threats (what issues exist that could negatively affect the company's situation). An SWOT analysis is both an external and an internal analysis of a company's current situation. Table 11.4 outlines an SWOT analysis of a hospital that is interested in opening a home healthcare agency.

This SWOT analysis is unique because of the role of HRM in the strategic planning. For example, there are seven typical strengths identified for a healthcare organization.

Table 11.4 SWOT Analysis: Healthcare Organization

Strengths	Weaknesses
Reputation	Competitive market
Accreditation	Leadership turnover (HRM)
Employee satisfaction (HRM)	Medicare reimbursement issues
Patient satisfaction	No management succession plan
Location	(HRM)
Award-winning services (HRM)	Weak strategic plan (HRM)
High occupancy rate	New healthcare legislation
Opportunities	**Threats**
Merge with other healthcare facilities (HRM)	Increased competition
	New technology adaptation
Purchase another facility	Labor shortages (HRM)
Improve information technology (HRM)	Economy
	Financial issues
Expand patient services	Accreditation issues
	Employee issues (HRM)

Of the seven, two—award-winning services and employee satisfaction—are a direct result of the positive role HRM plays in an organization, as the HR department provides training for the employees. Of the six identified weaknesses, leadership turnover, no management succession plan, and weak strategic plan all are a result of weak HRM. The HR department can turn these weaknesses into strengths by improving the selection plan for hiring employees and by working with senior management to develop a succession plan and a strategic plan for the organization. There were four opportunities identified, of which HRM could assist with two: information technology training for employees to improve efficiency and assistance with counseling of employees during a merger with another facility. Finally, of the seven threats identified, the HR department could help the organization manage labor shortages by training employees for job rotation and could train senior management on how to deal with employee issues. HRM can play a positive and integral role in strategic planning.

Based on the macroenvironment analysis, Porter's Five Forces analysis, and the SWOT analysis, it appears that starting a home healthcare agency could be beneficial to the hospital. Even if it is determined that the strengths and opportunities of the organization are positive, in order to ensure that this new venture is successful, the weaknesses of and threats to this hospital cannot be ignored and must be addressed in order to proceed.

■ Strategy Execution

Based on the SWOT, macroenvironment, and Porter's Five Forces analyses, the next step is to execute the strategy. **Strategy execution** is the most difficult step in the strategic management process because management is converting plans into actions. Executing the chosen strategy occurs at every level of the organization. To execute the strategy to achieve the desired objectives, the following must occur:

1. Employees must have the required skills and knowledge to implement the strategy.
2. There must be adequate financial resources allocated to strategy execution.
3. The infrastructure of the organization must support strategic implementation.
4. Employees must be motivated to execute the strategy. Tying incentives to productivity to achieve the strategy is an option.
5. The importance of strategy execution must be routinely communicated at all organizational levels (Thompson et al., 2012).

The Role of HRM in Strategy Execution: High-Performance Work System of a Healthcare Organization

From a strategic perspective, senior management should consider the formulation of a **high-performance work system**, which consists of the appropriate employees, technology, and structure that are put in place for strategy execution. Research has indicated this type of system recruits more job candidates, is more selective in its hiring process, and spends more hours providing employee training (Dessler, 2012).

According to Noe, Hollenbeck, Gerhart, and Wright (2011), **high-performance work system characteristics** consist of the following listed items. Any healthcare organization can use all of these system components. The role of HRM in the process is explained.

1. Employees work as a team: The concept of teamwork is common in the healthcare industry. Patients often require a team of providers for treatment. The HR department will provide training to employees on how to work well in teams.

2. Employees participate in selection of other employees: If nurses need to be hired, existing nurses should be included in the review of résumés and should participate in the interview process. They are familiar with the job responsibilities and can be intuitive about who would be successful in the organization. The HR department will develop a process for employee selection and will train employees on how to interview and how to select employees.

3. Formal performance feedback is an active process: A performance feedback system must be implemented in a timely manner, and feedback must be taken seriously by all parties. To improve employee performance, feedback must be considered. In conjunction with management, the HR department will develop a feedback system that is appropriate for the healthcare organization.

4. Employee rewards are linked to organizational performance: Healthcare organizations can link employee performance to healthcare quality indicators developed by the Agency for Healthcare Quality and Research such as prevention quality indicators, inpatient quality indicators, and patient safety quality indicators (Quality Indicators, 2011). The HR department will provide training to assess these types of metrics.

5. Technology is used to maximize processes: The organization must be scientifically current with any recent technologic advancement that can improve patient safety and care and that can improve organizational processes. For example, electronic health records are becoming a priority for health care. The HR department would coordinate training programs to ensure that this technology is used correctly by appropriate employees.

6. Ethical behavior is encouraged: The HR department will provide ethical training to all employees and will develop a code of conduct that is actively used with enforcement if unethical behavior occurs.

7. Employees must understand the importance of their jobs to the organization: The HR department will provide training to employees regarding their understanding of the importance of their roles in the organization. If employees feel empowered, their performance will be at a higher level.

8. Employees participate in any process or equipment changes: In conjunction with senior management, if there are changes that occur in an organization, the employees must be asked for input regarding any changes. If they believe their jobs are not challenging, then the HR department will change the job design or create different goals for the employees.

■ Strategy Evaluation

Once the strategy is executed, the final phase of strategic management is **strategy evaluation** by reviewing financial and strategic objectives. Strategy evaluation is the appraisal of plans and their results. According to Rumelt (1999), the strategy must be consistent with the mission, demonstrate a competitive advantage, and emphasize the strengths of the organization. If these objectives are met, then the strategy should be monitored to ensure there is no change in the external environment or within the competitive landscape. If the objectives established are not met, then the strategy must be reviewed for changes. The process of changing a strategy is the responsibility of senior management. The time frame for corrective action varies from days to months.

■ A Strategic Tool: Healthcare Workforce Planning

It is the responsibility of the HR department to review both existing and future labor needs of the organization. **Workforce planning** is the biannual or annual process of planning an organization's future job openings at all levels (Dessler, 2012). Workforce planning can be difficult due to the continued healthcare workforce shortages. As part of workforce planning, it is also necessary that the HR department assess rates for workforce shortages and internal workforce organizational changes due to employee turnover, layoffs, and any strategic changes. According to Soberg and Bennington (2009), several **HR metrics** that are analyzed include the following:

1. **Employee turnover rates:** Turnover can be both internal and external to the organization. Employees not only leave the organization through quitting, firing, and retirements but also transfer within departments. Each case should be analyzed.
2. **Leave of absence rates:** This metric includes maternity leave, disability, injuries, or illness.
3. **Productivity loss rate:** This metric can result from employee dissatisfaction or family illness, for example.
4. **Recruitment and selection rates:** How successful is the HR department in recruiting and selecting qualified employees?
5. **Organizational growth:** If the organization expands, how many employees will be needed?

Determining Labor Supply

Part of strategic forecasting is the assessment of both internal and external labor supply. Externally, it is important that economic and labor market conditions be analyzed to assess supply. The Congressional Budget Office and the Bureau of Labor Statistics provide economic projections and estimates of the availability of candidates for specific occupations (Dessler, 2012). As part of this process, the HR department performs a 5-year historical **trends analysis** to assess positive or negative trends. The HR department must also compare these rates with industry rates. If the organizational rates are below industry rates, no action may be needed. However, if the rates are above industry rates, then action must be taken.

Turnover rates in the healthcare industry occur at all employee levels: physicians, nurses, senior management, and administrative staff. Voluntary turnover (quitting) occurs with physicians and nurses because of professional disillusionment. This level of turnover can be devastating to an organization because there is a disruption in patient care, which could influence quality of care. Replacement of nonclinical staff has less of an impact. However, in a recent study of turnover impact on a major medical center, the annual cost of turnover for the center was 3.4% to 5.8% ($17 million to $20 million of its annual operating budget of $500 million). The largest replacement costs were the nursing staff. Recruitment costs for physician replacement was also very expensive (Waldman, Kelly, Arora & Smith, 2004).

By analyzing these metrics, the HR department can develop both short-term and long-term strategies to offset the negative trends. One of the most important HR metrics is recruitment rates. Successful recruitment and selection processes are crucial to ensure that qualified and appropriate employees are hired. If these processes do not occur, turnover rates will negatively affect productivity rates. In addition to the analysis of recruitment and selection rates, productivity rates related to job dissatisfaction are analyzed. If employees are dissatisfied, their performance will suffer. The HR department develops strategies to address employee dissatisfaction. Strategy development occurs by surveying employees routinely to determine workplace issues.

If an organization decides to increase healthcare services, a **ratio analysis** is performed to assess the number of employees that will be needed to satisfy the increased services (Mathis & Jackson, 2006). For example, if a hospital decided to add two new pediatric care floors, it will need to determine the ratio of registered nurses (RNs) to patients and the support staff needed per floor. If there will be 24 patients per floor with a ratio of 1 RN per 8 patients, the organization will be required to hire 3 RNs per floor for a total of 6 RNs. In addition to the actual wages paid, payroll and unemployment taxes must also be calculated.

Dealing with Workforce Shortages

In 2010, the American Hospital Association issued a report, *Workforce 2015: Strategy Trumps Shortages*, with the following recommendations:

1. Redesign work processes and use technology to increase efficiency and employee satisfaction.
2. Attract a new generation of workers by introducing a flexible organizational culture.
3. Retain existing workers by offering different incentives.
4. Train employees to be successful in teams.
5. Collaborate with educational institutions regarding their traditional degree programs to meet new work models, new technology, and critical thinking skills (American Hospital Association, 2010).

Dealing with labor shortages is a challenge for healthcare organizations. The HR department and management must develop an organizational culture that offers flexibility for work–life balance, encourages employee empowerment, is a leader in change, offers professional development for employees' careers and training to enhance their job performance, and encourages quality performance by offering incentives. These strategies will increase employee retention and performance, which will also lower employee turnover.

Budgeting

Labor expenses are the highest operating cost in an organization, particularly in health care, because of the high salaries of physicians and other healthcare providers. In addition, the healthcare industry is a service industry, which means that there will be high labor costs; therefore, the HR department must budget for labor costs. The salary budget typically consists of expenses associated with the salaries and wages of the employees. These expenses include benefits such as healthcare insurance, vacation, sick leave, and other benefits offered by the organization. A **labor budget** should predict the following: staffing levels, salaried versus wage employees, labor expenses such as overtime, benefits such as paid time off and health insurance, and taxes such as payroll taxes and unemployment taxes (Fried & Fottler, 2008). If an organization offers monetary incentives, this must also be included in the budget.

If an organization has determined that it does not have employees that can perform in an area of expertise, the organization will outsource the activity. **Outsourcing,** which consists of hiring an individual(s) external to the organization, is becoming more prevalent in healthcare information technology because of its rapid changes and its increased use in daily activities. If the organization determines that there are no employees who can provide a quality performance in a certain knowledge area, it will outsource the activity to an external individual. Outsourcing can be a cost-saving measure because the organization typically does not pay for the individual's benefits, thus decreasing substantial labor costs. A disadvantage of outsourcing activities is the potential lack of loyalty between the parties, as the outsourced individual is not truly part of the organization. If an organization outsources activities, the HR department should provide an orientation about the organization to the individual so the person can develop loyalty to the organization.

Succession Planning

If the departure of a CEO from an organization is unplanned, it can create an organization without direction. As part of strategic planning, a succession plan needs to be developed to ensure there is leadership continuity in the organization. **Succession planning** consists of a strategic plan that identifies replacements for key employees such as a CEO. However, in a healthcare organization, it is just as important to identify key replacements for lower-level employees such as the information technology executive, laboratory technicians, physical therapists, or other knowledge workers (Mathis & Jackson, 2006). In conjunction with management, the HR department should develop a plan to address the replacement of these key workers.

■ Conclusion

Strategic thinking is the ability to assess the organization's operations with a long-term perspective (Moseley, 2009). HRM plays an integral role in strategic management of any organization, including healthcare organizations. In order for a healthcare organization to be competitive, it must provide quality care to its consumers, or patients. Quality care comes from quality employees. Quality employees come from quality HRM procedures, which include a recruitment and selection process that will find the appropriate employees for an organization. The HR department must provide appropriate training for employees as healthcare organizations evolve and change their strategic plans. Long-term planning also requires employees to remain up to date with the newest scientific information regarding health care.

Employee turnover in a healthcare organization is very costly. The HR department can play a role in developing an organizational culture that empowers employees and encourages their productivity. Another integral role that the HR department plays in strategic planning is forecasting the supply of labor and the future labor demands of the healthcare organization. In addition to finding qualified employees for the organization, budgeting for labor costs is necessary because labor costs are the greatest operating expense of a healthcare organization.

■ Vocabulary

Advances in technology

Attractiveness of an industry

Balanced scorecard approach

Barriers to entry

Buyer forces' power

Competition

Demographic influences

Economic influences

Employee turnover
Employee turnover rates
Financial objectives
High-performance work system
High-performance work system
  characteristics
HR metrics
Human capital metrics
Labor budget
Leave of absence rates
Macroenvironment
Mission statement
Organizational growth
Outsourcing
Porter's Five Forces analysis
Productivity loss rate
Quality

Ratio analysis
Recruitment and selection rates
Sociocultural influences
Strategy evaluation
Strategic management
Strategic objectives
Strategic thinking
Strategy
Strategy execution
Substitute products or services
Succession plan
Suppliers
SWOT analysis
Trends analysis
Vision statement
Workforce planning

■ References

American Hospital Association (2010). *Workforce 2015: Strategy Trumps Shortages*. Available at: http://www.aha.org/aha/issues/Workforce/workforce2015.html. Accessed May 21, 2011.

Balanced Scorecard Basics (2011). Available at: http://www.balancedscorecard.org/BSCResources/AbouttheBalancedScorecard/tabid/55/Default.aspx. Accessed September 17, 2011.

Centers for Disease Control and Prevention (2011). Vision, Mission, Core Values, and Pledge: CDC Mission. Last updated January 11, 2011. Available at: http://www.cdc.gov/about/organization/mission.htm. Accessed December 1, 2011.

Dessler, G. (2012). *Fundamentals of Human Resource Management*. Upper Saddle River, NJ: Prentice Hall, pp. 54–56.

Duke Human Resources (2011). Balanced Scorecard. Available at: http://www.hr.duke.edu/managers/performance/DUHS/goals/scorecard.php. Accessed September 17, 2011.

Federal Emergency Management Agency (2011). About FEMA: What We Do. Last modified November 14, 2011. Available at: http://www.fema.gov/about/. Accessed December 1, 2011.

Fried, B. & Fottler, M. (2008). *Human Resources in Healthcare* (3rd ed.). Chicago, IL: Health Administration Press, pp. 11–12.

Graham, J. & Havlick, W. (1994). *Mission Statements: A Guide to the Corporate and Nonprofit Sectors*. New York, NY: Garland Publishing, pp. 1–8.

Hader, R. (2006). More than words: Provide a clear and concise mission statement. Available at: http://www.nursingmanagement.com. Accessed May 22, 2011.

Institute of Medicine (1998). Measuring the quality of health care. Available at: http://www.iom.edu/Reports/1998/Measuring-the-Quality-of-Health-Care.aspx. Accessed January 1, 2012.

Inyang, B. (2010). Strategic human resource management (SHRM): A paradigm for achieving sustained competitive advantage in organization. *International Bulletin of Business Administration*, 7:23–36.

Mathis, R. & Jackson, J. (2006). *Human Resource Management* (11th ed.). Mason, OH: Thomson/South-Western, pp. 17–19.

Moseley, G., (2009). Managing Health Care Business Strategy. Sudbury, MA: Jones and Bartlett Publishers, p. 11.

Noe, R., Hollenbeck, J., Gerhart, B. & Wright, P. (2011). *Fundamentals of Human Resource Management* (3rd ed.). New York, NY: McGraw-Hill/Irwin, pp. 128–129.

Porter, M. E. (1979). How competitive forces shape strategy. *Harvard Business Review*, 57(March–April):86–93.

Quality Indicators (2011). Available at: http://www.qualityindicators.ahrq.org. Accessed May 23, 2011.

Rumelt, R. (1999). Notes on strategy evaluation. Available at: http://www.anderson.ucla.edu/faculty/dick.rumelt/Docs/Notes/StratEvaluation1999.pdf. Accessed October 2, 2011.

Soberg, A. & Bennington, A. (2009). Workforce planning: Implications for healthcare in Canada and elsewhere. *People & Strategy*, 32(3):27–32.

Tellez, M. (2011). Why patients prefer home health. Available at: http://blog.medistarhomehealth.com/2011/07/07/why-patients-prefer-home-health/. Accessed September 28, 2011.

Thompson, A., Peteraf, M., Gamble, J. & Strickland, A. (2012). *Crafting & Executing Strategy: The Quest for Competitive Advantage* (18th ed.). Boston, MA: McGraw-Hill/Irwin, pp. 1–15, 30.

Thompson, A., Strickland, A. & Gamble, J. (2010). *Crafting & Executing Strategy: The Quest for Competitive Advantage* (17th ed.). Boston, MA: McGraw-Hill/Irwin, pp. 1–15.

U.S. Unemployment Rate (2011). Available at: http://www.tradingeconomics.com/united-states/unemployment-rate. Accessed September 16, 2011.

Waldman, J., Kelly, F., Arora, S. & Smith, H. (2004). The shocking cost of turnover in healthcare. *Healthcare Management Review*, 29(1):2–7.

STUDENT WORKBOOK ACTIVITY 11.1

Complete the following case scenarios based on the information provided in this chapter. You must use two vocabulary or key terms discussed in the text in each of your four answers. You can repeat two terms once.

Real-Life Applications: Case Scenario 1

You are working for a skilled nursing facility. Your manager is concerned because of the high turnover in nurses. Several of the nurses have gone to other facilities. She has asked you to find out why there is such a high turnover rate.

Activity

She has asked that you develop a plan that will increase employee satisfaction. Using the Internet and text, develop a long range plant to develop motivational strategies to reduce employee turnover.

Responses

_____

_____

_____

_____

_____

Real-Life Applications: Case Scenario 2

Your hospital is planning on opening a pediatric floor. It is anticipated that there will be 24 pediatric patients on the floor. Your boss has asked you to project the labor needed for this floor.

Activity

Develop a projected labor budget. Research the Internet to find out the cost of how much to pay the anticipated clinical staff.

Responses

_____

_____

_____

_____

Real-Life Applications: Case Scenario 3

The CEO of your healthcare network is interested in expanding to other services. The network is trying to determine if it should open an emergent care facility in the area. There are currently four other such facilities. She has asked your opinion on this option.

Activity

Perform Porter's Five Forces analysis for this project and provide a recommendation as to whether the network should proceed with this new center.

Responses

_____

_____

_____

_____

Real-Life Applications: Case Scenario 4

The CEO of HealthyAreUs Hospital believes that employees are not performing to their best ability. Other hospitals are considered a great place to work, and employees are happy there and are very productive. He has heard the term "high-performance organization" and wants HealthyAreUs to become one.

Activity

Research information on high-performance organizations and provide five methods that could be used to improve productivity at HealthyAreUs.

Responses

_____

_____

_____

_____

_____

STUDENT WORKBOOK ACTIVITY 11.2

In Your Own Words

Please describe these core concepts in your own words.

Vision statement:

_____

_____

_____

_____

Strategic management:

_____

_____

_____

_____

Outsourcing:

_____

_____

_____

_____

High-performance organization:

_____

_____

_____

_____

Workforce planning:

_____

_____

_____

_____

Labor budget:

_____

_____

_____

_____

Quality:

_____

_____

_____

_____

Trends analysis:

_____

_____

_____

_____

Ratio analysis:

_____

_____

_____

_____

Mission statement:

_____

_____

_____

_____

STUDENT WORKBOOK ACTIVITY 11.3

Internet Exercises

Write your answers in the spaces provided.

- Visit each of the websites that are listed in the text that follows.
- Name the organization.
- Locate its mission statement on its website. If the organization does not have a mission statement, describe its purpose.
- Apply this organization to the chapter information.

Websites
http://www.nursingmanagement.com

Organization name:

_____

Mission statement:

_____

_____

_____

Overview of activities:

_____

_____

_____

Application to chapter information:

_____

_____

_____

http://www.qualityindicators.ahrq.gov

Organization name:

_____

Mission statement:

_____

_____

_____

Overview of activities:

_____

_____

_____

Application to chapter information:

_____

_____

_____

http://www.kmworld.com

Organization name:

_____

Mission statement:

_____

_____

_____

Overview of activities:

_____

_____

_____

Application to chapter information:

_____

_____

_____

http://www.healthcareitnews.com
Organization name:

_____

Mission statement:

_____

_____

_____

Overview of activities:

_____

_____

_____

Application to chapter information:

_____

_____

_____

http://www.aacn.org
Organization name:

_____

Mission statement:

_____

_____

_____

Overview of activities:

_____

_____

_____

Application to chapter information:

_____

_____

_____

http://www.hrhresourcecenter.org
Organization name:

_____

Mission statement:

_____

_____

_____

Overview of activities:

_____

_____

_____

Application to chapter information:

_____

_____

_____

STUDENT ACTIVITY 11.4: DISCUSSION BOARDS FOR ONLINE, HYBRID, AND TRADITIONAL ONGROUND CLASSES

Discussion Board Guidelines

The discussion board is used in online and web-enhanced courses in place of classroom lectures and discussion. The board can be an enhancement to traditional classes. The discussion board is the way in which the students "link together" as a class. The following are guidelines to help focus on the discussion topic and to define the roles and responsibilities of the discussion coordinator and other members of the class. The educator will be the discussion moderator for this course.

1. The educator will post the discussion topic and directions for the upcoming week. These postings should all be responses to the original topic or responses to other students' responses. When people respond to what someone else has posted, they should start the posting with the person's name so it is clear which

message they are responding to. **A response such as "Yes" or "I agree" does not count for credit. Your responses must be in your own words. You cannot copy and paste from the text.**

2. Postings (especially responses) should include enough information so the message is clear but should not be so long that it becomes difficult to follow. Remember, this is like talking to someone in a classroom setting. The postings should reflect the content of the text or other assignments. If you retrieve information from the Internet, the hyperlink must be cited.

3. Students should check the discussion daily to see if new information has been posted that requires their attention and response.

Good discussion will often include different points of view. Students should feel free to disagree or "challenge" others to support their positions or ideas. All discussions must be handled in a respectful manner. The following are discussion boards for this chapter.

Discussion Boards

1. What is strategic management? How does that apply to the healthcare industry? Be specific.

2. Give examples of the macroenvironment. How do they apply to the healthcare industry?

3. What is a SWOT analysis? How would that process be beneficial to a healthcare organization?

4. List three characteristics of a high-performance work system in a healthcare organization. Be specific. How can HRM play a role in this process?

INDEX

Note: Tables are noted with *t*.

CPR. *See* Cardiopulmonary resuscitation
Credentialing examination, 143
Criminal background checks, 116
Criminal law, 34
Criterion validity, 118
Criticism, careful, 221
Cross-cultural competencies, employee training in, 13
CTO. *See* Chief technology officer
Cultural awareness training, 217–218
Cultural competency, 285
  equitable health care and, 286
Cultural competency model, 285–286
Culturally competent, defined, 217
Culturally competent healthcare organizations, guidelines for, 285–286
Cytotechnologists, 153

D

Dana-Farber Cancer Institute, vision statement for, 318, 319*t*
da Vinci Surgical System, 293
Decision model for healthcare dilemmas, 51–53
Defensive medicine, 35
Defined benefit plans, 189
Defined contribution plans, 189
Demographic influences, 322
Demographic trends, in workforce and population, 13
Dental Admission Test, 151
Dental assistants, 148
Dental hygienists, 148, 152
Dental insurance, 187, 193
Dental schools, accredited, 148
Dentists, 10, 142, 148
Department of Labor. *See* U.S. Department of Labor
Dependent care accounts, 191
Developmental psychologists, 150
Development and training programs, employee motivation and, 11
Diagnostic medical sonographers, 153–154
Dictionary of Occupational Titles, 85
Dieticians, 152

Dignity, ethics in healthcare industry and, 50
Direct methods of recruiting, 110
Directors of physical therapy, training or experience for, 7–8
Disability insurance, 178, 179*t*, 193
  long-term, 187–188
  short-term, 188
Disabled persons, legislative protection for, 39, 42
Disabled workers, prohibiting discrimination against, 5*t*
Disaster-specific policies, 183
Discipline of employees, 265–266
Discrimination
  avoiding issues of, 117
  EEOC and processing complaints related to, 47
  legislative prohibition against, 39
Disparate impact, 123, 124*t*
Disparate treatment, 123
Disparities of access to health care, addressing, 13
Distance learning programs, 216
Distributive justice, 211
Diversity in healthcare workforce, 283–300
  hiring practices, 122–123
  increasing, 284–286
  training programs for, 217–218
Diversity of workforce (in general)
  affirmative action plan and, 48
  demographics and trends in, 13
DO. *See* Doctor of osteopathic medicine
Doctor of chiropractic degree, 149
Doctor of medicine, 142, 143
Doctor of osteopathic medicine, 142, 143
Doctor of podiatric medicine, 151
Doctor of psychology, 151
Doctor-patient relationship, codes of ethics and, 53–54
Doctors Council, 245
Doctors of optometry, 149
DOT. *See* Dictionary of Occupational Titles
Drug Free Workplace Act of 1988, 41
Drug use, risk profiles for, 114
Due process methods, 263–265

Duke University Health System (DUHS)
  balanced scorecard for, 320, 320*t*
  Peking University agreement with, 288
DVDs, 216

E

EBS. *See* Employee Benefits Survey
Economic and Social Council (UN), 111
Economic influences, 321
Education, reimbursement for, 191, 193
Educational recruitment, at job fairs, 109–110
Education and training
  for anesthesiologist assistants, 152–153
  for cardiovascular technologists, 153
  for certified midwives, 147
  for certified nurse midwives, 147
  for chiropractors, 149
  for clinical laboratory technologists, 160–161
  for dentists, 148
  for electroneurodiagnostic technologists, 154
  for EMTs, 155
  for exercise scientists, 155
  for exercises physiologists, 155
  for health services administrators, 159
  for kinesiotherapists, 155
  for licensed practical nurses, 145
  for medical illustrators, 156
  for nuclear medicine technologists, 160
  for nurse practitioners, 146
  for optometrists, 149
  for orthotists and prosthetists, 156
  for perfusionists, 156
  for personal fitness trainers, 157
  for pharmacists, 148
  for physician assistants, 144–145
  for physicians, 142–143
  for podiatrists, 151
  for polysomnographic technologists, 157
  for psychologists, 151

for radiation therapists, 159
for registered nurses, 145–146
for respiratory therapists, 157
for surgeon technologists, 158
for surgical assistants, 158
EEOC. *See* Equal Employment Opportunity Commission
EEO-1 reports, 48
Effective workforce, human resource management and, 4
Efficiency, 15
eflexgroup, 192
EHRs. *See* Electronic health records
ejobfairs.net, 110
Eldercare, 190–191, 193
Electroneurodiagnostic technologists, 154
Electronic health records, 284, 289–292
benefits of, 290–292
competency model, 86, *89*
defined, 289, 290
history behind, 289–290
Electronic job fairs, 110
Electronic job postings, 109, 113
Electronic job recruitment, diverse opportunities for, examples, 110
Electronic medical records, 289–292, 321
benefits of, 290–292
defined, 289
history behind, 289–290
Element, 82
Emergency medical service, 154
Emergency medical technicians-paramedics, 154–155
Emergency Unemployment Compensation program, 181
Emotional stability, 115
Employee analysis, 213
Employee appraisals, routine performance of, 221
Employee benefits, 11, 177–194
budgeting, 329
cafeteria plans, 192
childcare and eldercare, 190–191
education reimbursement, 191
family and medical leave, 177, 182
flexible work schedules, 191
group medical insurance, 182–186

life insurance, 187–188
long-term care insurance, 186
paid vacation and sick leave, 189–190
as recruitment tool, 177
retirement plans, 188–189
selecting, 192
social security, 177, 178–179
unemployment insurance, 177, 179, 181
workers' compensation, 177, 181–182
Employee Benefits Survey, 192
Employee career development, 221
Employee development, 11
Employee discharge, 262
Employee discipline, 265–266
Employee dismissal, 262
Employee handbook, importance of, 266–267
Employee performance, 210
motivational strategies for, 212
training programs and, 212–213
Employee Retirement Income Security Act of 1974, 37*t*, 40, 189
Employees, 3
diverse, hiring, 122–123
empowerment of, 221
fair selection processes for, 123
motivating, 210–212
rights and responsibilities of, 261–262
terminating, 12–13
training and development for, 11, 247
Employee separation, types of, 262
Employee turnover, 328, 330
Employee turnover rates, 327
Employers, rights and responsibilities of, 261–262
Employment, defined, 261
Employment agencies
budgeting and, 113
private, 109
temporary services, 109
Employment-at-will doctrine, 262–263
Employment-at-will policies, exceptions to, 263
Employment practices liability insurance, 264, 265
Empowerment of employees, 221

EMRs. *See* Electronic medical records
EMS. *See* Emergency medical service
EMTs. *See* Emergency medical technicians-paramedics
End-of-life decisions, 219
EOPs. *See* Exclusive provider organizations
EPLI. *See* Employment practices liability insurance
e-prescribing, database elements for, 292
Equal Employment Opportunity Commission, 118, 123
creation of, 47
role of, 47–48
information and education, 48
issuing regulations, 47–48
processing complaints, 47
Equal employment opportunity employers, hiring diverse employees, 122–123
Equal opportunity employment, 39
Equal Pay Act of 1963, *5t*, 6, 36, 37*t*, 48
Equitable health care, cultural competency and, 286
Equity theory, 211, 221
Ergonomics
defined, 90
OSHA standards for, 49
ERISA. *See* Employee Retirement Income Security Act of 1974
Essential job functions, 42, 84
Ethical behavior, 33
Ethical issues, in health care, 8–9
Ethical standards, 49, 218
Ethics, 218–219
defined, 49–50
in healthcare workplace, basic concepts of, 49–51
in public health, 219
research and, 55–56
Exclusive provider organizations, 184
Exercise scientists, 155
Exercises physiologists, 155
Exit interview, termination of employees and, 268
Expectancy theory, 210–211, 220
Experience rating, 181
Experiential programs, 217

Interviewers
    characteristics of, 118, 120, 122
    diverse, 122
Interviews, 116–117
    behavioral, 116
    common questions during, 117t
    situational, 116
    structured, 116
    unstructured, 116–117
Intrinsic (or internal) rewards, 210,
        212, 221
Intuitive Surgical, 293
Invasion of privacy, 34–35
Involuntary termination, 266
IOM. *See* Institute of Medicine
IPAs. *See* Independent practice
        associations
IPE. *See* Interprofessional education
iPods, 216
IRBs. *See* Institutional review
        boards
IT. *See* Information technology

J

Jehovah's Witnesses, blood transfu-
        sions and, 50
Job analysis, 9, 93
    description of, 82–83
    importance of, 84
    performing, 83
Job analyst, role of, 83–84
Job design, 9, 90, 93
Job enlargement, 91, 93, 219, 220
Job enrichment, 11–12, 91, 93,
        219, 220
Job fairs, 109–110
Job hazard analysis technique, 218
Job identification, 90
Job Interview Assessment Rubric,
        119t
Job lock, 41
Job postings, 108, 120t
Job redesign, 11, 219–220
    examples of, 91
    flexible work schedules, 92
    job sharing, 92
    self-directed work teams, 91–92
    telework, 92
Job rotation, 91, 93, 219
Job schedule design, 9
Job sharing, 92, 93
Job specifications, 90
Joint Commission, 9, 59, 285, 297

Joint Commission International,
        287
Joint Review Committee on Educa-
        tion Programs in Nuclear
        Medicine Technology, 160
Justice, ethics in healthcare industry
        and, 50, 51

K

Kaiser Permanente, 285, 296
Kentucky River Community Care,
        Inc., 242
Kinesiotherapists, 155
Kinesiotherapy, defined, 155
Knowledge, skills, and abilities,
        and other characteristics
        (KSAs), 90–91, 210, 213,
        220

L

Laboratory technologists and tech-
        nicians, 11, 152, 209
Labor budget, 329
Labor supply, determining, 328
Labor unions, 238
    early history of, 4
    goal of, 6
    health care and, 12
Landrum-Griffin Act, 239
Language barriers, 285
Lateral violence, 57
Law
    civil, 34
    common, 34
    criminal, 34
    defined, 34
    healthcare workplace and basic
        concepts of, 34–35
Layoffs, 266
Leave of absence rates, 327
Ledbetter, Lilly, 45
Legal awareness training, 218
Legal issues, in health care, 8–9
Legally defensible, 10, 118
Legal ramifications of selection
        process, 118
Legislation, human resource-
        related, 37t–39t
Lehigh Valley Health Network
        (Pennsylvania), cultural
        competency model for,
        285

Licensed practical nurses, education
        for, 145
Licensing examinations, for physi-
        cians, 142
Licensure, for optometrists,
        149–150
Life expectancy
    increase in, 13
    long-term care insurance and rise
        in, 186
Life insurance, 187–188
Lifting patients, OSHA standards
        for, 49
Lilly Ledbetter Fair Pay Act of
        2009, 6t, 7, 39t, 45–46,
        48
Lincoln Financial Group, 188t
LinkedIn, healthcare organizations
        on, 110, 111
Local government job openings,
        websites for, 109
Long-term care, supports, and ser-
        vices competency model,
        86, 88
Long-term care insurance, 186, 193
Long-term disability insurance,
        187–188
LPNs. *See* Licensed practical nurses

M

Macroenvironment analysis,
        320–322
    demographic influences, 322
    economic influences, 321
    governmental and legal influ-
        ences, 321
    sociocultural influences, 321–322
    technologic influences, 321
Mail order pharmacies, 148
Major medical policies, 183
Malpractice insurance premiums,
        increase in, 35
Managed care organizations, 183,
        244
Managed care plans, 183
Management by objectives, 221
Management competencies, 86
Management Position Description
        Questionnaire, 83
Management transparency, 221
Mandatory benefits, 11
Massachusetts Nurses Association,
        238, 244

Vision coverage, 187, 193
Vision statements
  development of, 317–318
  for healthcare organizations,
    318, 319*t*
  role of, 316
Voluntary benefits, 11, 182
Voluntary hospitals, 36
VR. *See* Virtual reality

W

Wages, for unionized *vs.* non-union
  workers, 239. *See also*
  Salaries
Wagner Act. *See* National Labor
  Relations Act (Wagner
  Act)
Walgreens, on-site health clinics
  at, 185
Walt Disney Parks and Resorts, on-
  site health clinics at, 185
Webinars, 216
Websites, electronic job postings
  on, 109
Wellstone Act, 44
Weyco, smoking ban and, 263
White Memorial Medical Center
  (Los Angeles), cultural
  competency model for,
  285

Whole-life insurance, 187
Women
  anti-discrimination legislation
    and, 48
  in health care workforce, 13
  increased workforce participa-
    tion by, 190
  senior healthcare management
    and underrepresentation
    of, 284
Work activity, 82
Worker Adjustment and Retraining
  Notification Act of 1989,
  37*t*, 42
Workers' compensation, 177,
  181–182, 193
Workflow analysis, 82
*Workforce 2015: Strategy Trumps
  Shortages*, 328
Workforce planning, 327
Workforce shortages, dealing with,
  328–329
Working mothers, labor rate for,
  190
Work-life balance, 329
Workplace bullying
  awareness training, 8
  different terms for, 56
  eliminating, recommendation for,
    58–59
  in health care, 57

impact of, 58
  as international issue, 56–59
  legal implications of, 58
  prevalence of, 56–57
Workplace Bullying Institute
  establishment of, 57
  Healthy Workplace Bill, 59
Workplace competencies, 86
Workplace diversity, defined,
  284. *See also* Diversity in
  healthcare workforce
Workplace hazards, OSHA and,
  48–49
Workplace violence, risk profiles
  for, 114
Work samples, 123
World War I, 6
Wrongful discharge, 263

Y

YouTube, 15, 216, 299